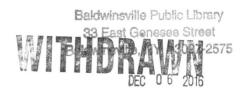

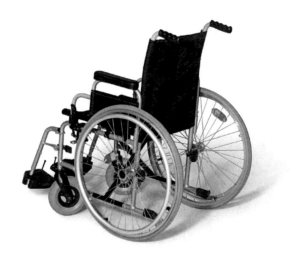

THE EMPTY CHAIR

A Movement to
Limit the Wheelchair
and Lead a Healthy Life

Howard B. Cotler MD, FACS, FAAOS, FABOS

THE EMPTY CHAIR: *A Movement to Limit the Wheelchair and Lead a Healthy Life*

DEC 0 6 2016

Published by Atlantic Publishing Group, Inc.
1405 SW 6th Avenue • Ocala, Florida 34471 • Phone 800-814-1132 • Fax 352-622-1875
Website: www.atlantic-pub.com • Email: sales@atlantic-pub.com
SAN Number: 268-1250

Library of Congress Cataloging-in-Publication Data
Names: Cotler, H. B. (Howard B.), author.
Title: The empty chair : a movement to limit the wheelchair and lead a
    healthy life / by Howard Cotler MD, FACS, FAAOS, FABOS?E.
Description: Ocala, Florida : Atlantic Publishing Group, Inc., [2016] |
    Includes bibliographical references and index.
Identifiers: LCCN 2016002472| ISBN 9781620231357 (alk. paper) | ISBN 1620231352 (alk. paper)
Subjects: LCSH: Wheelchairs. | People with disabilities.
Classification: LCC RD757.W4 C68 2016 | DDC 617/.033--dc23 LC record available at http://lccn.loc.gov/2016002472

Cover Design: Jackie Miller
Interior Design: Meg Buchner • megadesn@mchsi.com

Printed in the United States

Reduce. Reuse.
RECYCLE.

A decade ago, Atlantic Publishing signed the Green Press Initiative. These guidelines promote environmentally friendly practices, such as using recycled stock and vegetable-based inks, avoiding waste, choosing energy-efficient resources, and promoting a no-pulping policy. We now use 100-percent recycled stock on all our books. The results: in one year, switching to post-consumer recycled stock saved 24 mature trees, 5,000 gallons of water, the equivalent of the total energy used for one home in a year, and the equivalent of the greenhouse gases from one car driven for a year.

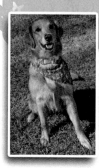 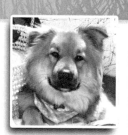 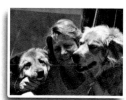

Over the years, we have adopted a number of dogs from rescues and shelters. First there was Bear and after he passed, Ginger and Scout. Now, we have Kira, another rescue. They have brought immense joy and love not just into our lives, but into the lives of all who met them.

We want you to know a portion of the profits of this book will be donated in Bear, Ginger and Scout's memory to local animal shelters, parks, conservation organizations, and other individuals and nonprofit organizations in need of assistance.

– Douglas & Sherri Brown,
President & Vice-President of Atlantic Publishing

DEDICATIONS

Florence Dion Cotler
who nurtured two spine surgeons

Jerome M. Cotler MD
a mentor and father

Paul R. Meyer Jr. MD
a mentor and second father

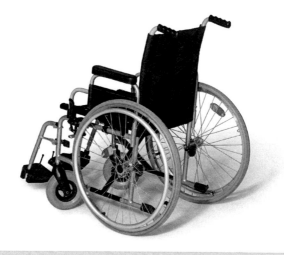

TABLE OF CONTENTS

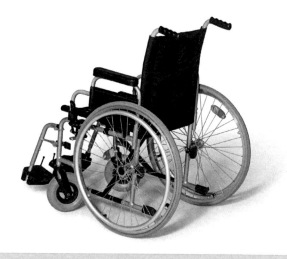

INTRODUCTION

C urrently one out of every hundred people in the United States is wheelchair dependent. This has created a huge personal and financial burden on those individuals, their families, the government and society as a whole.

When thinking of wheelchair usage, most people immediately think of those with paralysis from a spinal condition such as Christopher Reeve or Governor Greg Abbott. But the most common reasons for wheelchair use are actually stroke and osteoarthritis. Chronic serious back problems are another major cause. Additionally, chronic conditions such as multiple sclerosis, obesity, cancer, closed head injury, polytrauma and simply being elderly provide additional wheelchair needs. The disease of in

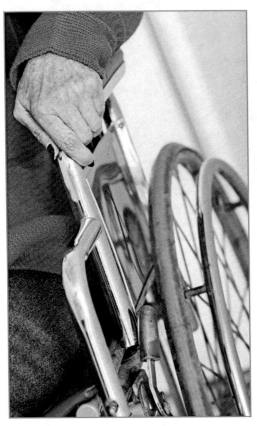

activity resulting from any one of these injuries or illnesses oftentimes results in wheelchair dependency. Through activity-based exercise programs, nutrition programs and careful symptomatic care this exacerbation of the disease process may be avoided. All this needs to be considered while undergoing care for your primary diagnosis.

Wheelchairs are, unfortunately, a visible sign of disability, at least as perceived by the public and sometimes by the user. There is a certain percentage of wheelchair users that will never be able to walk again. But if prevention, earlier intervention, more aggressive self-help and exercise programs were utilized more often there would be far fewer wheelchair users. By taking better care of yourself now, you may prevent the need for a wheelchair later.

Like my father before me, I have dedicated my life and career to helping those who have suffered. So for the past 30 years as a practicing orthopedic surgeon specializing in spine care, I have tried to eradicate paralysis and dysfunction — both physically and mentally — and return people back to leading active and productive lives.

My journey began as a son of an orthopedic surgeon who was a co-founder of Delaware Valley Regional SCI Center, one of the 14 regional spinal cord injury model systems. I subsequently had the privilege of training in three of the model centers and worked in one for 17 years. Through this battlefield education I have come to appreciate how precious and fragile life is — a delicate balance between normal and chaos.

My awakening came one day when I was riding my bike and, after hitting a crack in the road, flipped over the handlebars. I was not wearing a helmet and came to the immediate fear of sustaining a spinal cord injury. Here I was, a young orthopedic surgeon with a young family who, in an instant, could have become paralyzed by a freak accident. I was given a second chance. Many are not so fortunate. From that day forward I knew that I had a calling — to treat patients with spinal disorders and educate patients, families and the public on injuries and their prevention. And if improvement is not possible, then my goal is to give my patient the hope and self-confidence to choose ability over disability. We are forever hopeful that eventually some or all wheelchair users will be able to walk again.

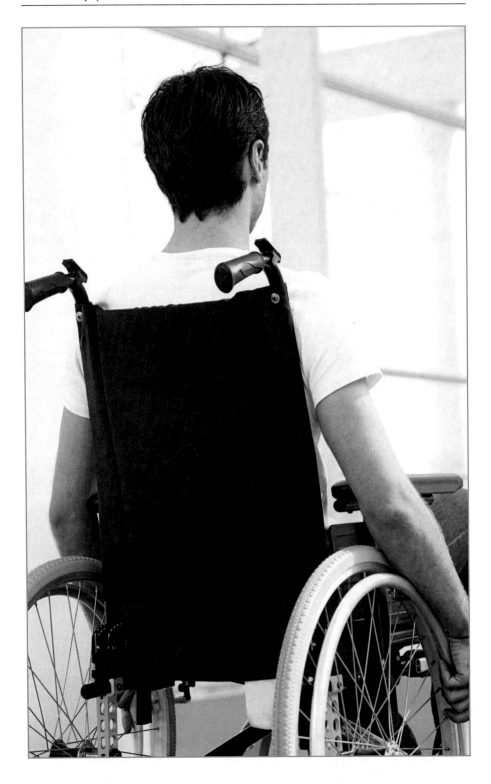

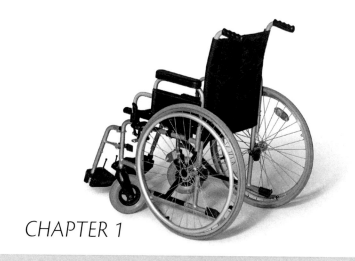

CHAPTER 1

ANATOMY

There are two very important anatomical systems to consider when dealing with paralysis. The first is the nervous system, which coordinates voluntary and involuntary actions, and transmits signals to and receives signals from various parts of the body. The brain and spinal cord are the command center, or the central nervous system. From the command center the spinal cord conveys messages, or impulses, to and from the peripheral nerves (both motor and sensory), which allows the extremities to function. The command center also sends messages to the autonomic nerves, which control the vital organs.

The second system is the musculoskeletal system, which is concerned with locomotion. The musculoskeletal system consists of the axial spine and the extremities. The spine consists of blocks of bone that stack up one on top of another and are separated by discs. These discs act as the shock absorbers of the skeleton and have the consistency of crabmeat. The extremities consist of bones, muscles, ligaments, vessels and nerves, which are for useful function (locomotion, activities of daily living, vocation, etc.).

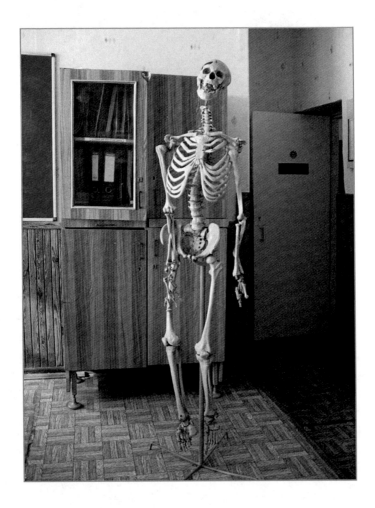

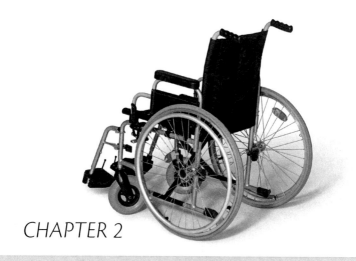

CHAPTER 2

INCIDENCE

n 2011, approximately 5.5 million people sustained some form of paralysis. The majority was from stroke (29 percent), but spinal cord injury (23 percent) and multiple sclerosis (17 percent) accounted for a significant portion of the conditions as well. Over 60 percent of those paralyzed are under 40 years of age. Motor vehicle accidents, industrial accidents and falls accounted for the majority of spinal cord injuries.

This young, previously healthy population is stricken in their prime productive years and faced with a life-altering occurrence. How they and their families navigate this diagnosis sets the stage for the rest of their lives.

More than one third of the American population is obese. Obesity-related conditions, including heart disease, stroke, cancer and Type II diabetes, are the leading causes of preventable deaths.

Osteoarthritis is the most common joint disorder in the United States. Osteoarthritis is a multifactorial disease where the most common causes are aging, obesity, previous joint injury, muscle weakness and weight-bearing intolerance. Symptomatic osteoarthritis is defined by the presence of pain, aching or stiffness of a joint with associated radiographic findings. These symptoms may apply to the hip, knee, spine and/or any extremity joint. It is hard to determine the specific incidence of osteoarthritis, but in one study, symptomatic osteoarthritis of the knee was found in approximately 40 percent of men and 47 percent of women. The incidence increases to 60 percent in those patients with a body mass index (BMI) of 30 or higher.

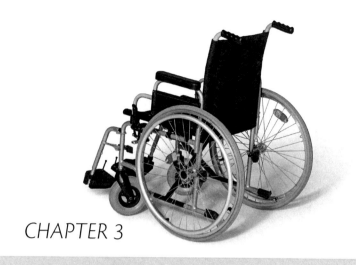

CHAPTER 3

COMMON CAUSES OF WHEELCHAIR USAGE

Osteopenia, Osteoporosis and Fragility Fractures

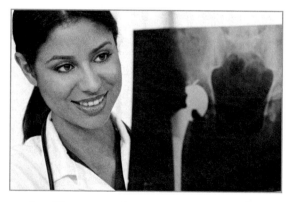

Osteopenia is a medical condition where bone mineral density is below normal, but not to the point of developing osteoporosis. The most common bone disease in humans is osteoporosis. Osteoporosis affects one in two women and one in five men older than 50 years in the United States. It is estimated that, among adults older than 50 years of age, more than 54 million have osteoporosis.

Approximately 2 million fragility fractures occur annually. The lifetime risk of osteoporotic fractures is about 40–50 percent in women and 13–22 percent in men. These fragility fractures result in pain, loss of function and deterioration of the quality of life.

Bone mineral density is determined by dual-energy X-ray absorptiometry (DXA, formerly DEXA). DXA gives a value called a T score; a T score of -1.0 or greater is normal, -1 to -2.5 is low bone mass or osteopenia, and -2.5 or below is osteoporosis.

The at-risk population for osteoporosis is thin, Caucasian women over 65 with a family history of osteoporosis and a history of long-term use of steroids or anticonvulsants, eating disorders or diseases, smoking, inactivity, excessive alcohol consumption, and diet low in calcium and vitamin D.

Generally, osteoporosis is asymptomatic. The diagnosis is often made after a fracture occurs. These fractures most commonly involve the wrist, hip and spine. Fractures that occur in these areas are due to the loss of sponge-like bone inside the outer shell of the bone. This loss of spongy bone usually begins between the ages of 30–35, and occurs to a higher degree in women. These fractures can result in pain and disability, deformity and early death.

The prevention of osteoporosis requires lifestyle changes — smoking cessation, moderate alcohol use, weight-bearing exercise, and calcium and vitamin D supplements. Additionally, fall prevention, balance preservation interventions, resistance exercise and optimization of serum vitamin D levels need to be considered.

Calcium and vitamin D daily recommendations

Adults under 50 and men 50-70: 1,000 mg of calcium and 400–800 IU of vitamin D

Women 51–70: 1,200 mg of calcium and 400–800 IU of vitamin D

Adults over 70: 1,200 mg of calcium and 800 IU of vitamin D

Supplementation with other medications, such as biphosphonates, teriparatide, raloxifene, and denosumab may be required after consultation with your family physician or internist. These anti-osteoporotic therapies reduce the risk of initial fragility fractures and prevent subsequent fragility fractures.

The season of heartburn often occurs around Thanksgiving time when people indulge in sweets with mint, chocolate and other triggers that result in acid reflux. Acid reflux is the most common gastrointestinal diagnosis, causing approximately 9 million visits to physicians in 2009 alone. In the late 1980s, a group of medications was introduced called proton pump inhibitors (PPI). These PPIs are commonly known as Prilosec OTC (Proctor & Gamble, Cincinnati), Nexium (AstraZeneca, London), Prevacid (Takeda Pharmaceuticals, Osaka, Japan), Dexilant (Takeda Pharmaceuticals, Osaka, Japan), AcipHex (Eisai Inc. Woodcliff Lake, New Jersey) and Protonix (Pfizer, New York). These medications, once started, often continue for the life of the patient. PPIs affect calcium metabolism by promoting accelerated loss of calcium from the bones and also impair the absorption of calcium from the diet. Thus these medications appear to increase the risk of osteoporosis, which also increases the risk of fracture. PPIs also impair the absorption of magnesium, interfere with the absorption of other nutrients, which may result in anemia, and may result in irritable bowel syndrome or hypermotility of the G.I. tract. So for those patients taking these medications, a closer monitoring of their calcium and vitamin D is needed.

Once a spinal fracture or fracture of a major weight-bearing bone occurs, the treatment of the fracture may be by either brace or surgery. After stabilization of the fracture, mobilization, weight-bearing exercise and medical management are needed. Subsequent safety evaluation and injury prevention strategies are essential to prevent additional injuries. It has been reported that only one in five adults with fragility fractures receive treatment after the first event. This lack of follow-up care may result in a compounding of the problem and the progression to continued weight-bearing intolerance.

Weight-Bearing Intolerance

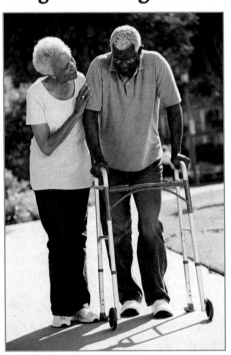

When a person develops an injury, illness or disease that does not allow them to stand and bear weight on their legs we say they have developed a weight-bearing intolerance. When a weight-bearing intolerance develops, people usually elect to use mobility aids such as canes, crutches or a walker to assist them in bearing weight so that they can continue to walk. If walking decreases and a mobility aid such as a wheelchair is used, then a vicious medical cycle occurs. This state of deconditioning and inactivity will affect many organ systems in what we call the **disease of inactivity**. The musculoskeletal system has the most obvious decline due to deconditioning and inactivity. A person can lose 10–20 percent of their muscle strength as a result of one week of inactivity and/or bed rest. The thigh muscle can lose 3 percent of its mass in one week. The greatest loss of muscle mass occurs in the back and the weight-bearing muscles of the legs. Osteoporosis, or soft bone, can occur when bones are not weight bearing. This situation has been commonly referred to as disuse osteoporosis. When bones are not being stressed or bearing weight, the bone cells take calcium out of the bones and place it in the bloodstream. This transfer of calcium can result in kidney stones. After three months of bed rest or inactivity bone density is approximately 50 percent less than normal. This decrease in bone density makes the bones more susceptible to fracture. With the occurrence of a fracture due to soft bone, the situation dramatically worsens the disease of inactivity, and the cycle remains unbroken. So how does one break the circle when pain and misery continue to chase each other?

DISEASE OF INACTIVITY

- Loss of muscle mass
- Disuse osteoporosis
- Kidney stones
- Pathologic fracture
- Cardiovascular disease
- Blood clots
- Pneumonia
- GI tract pathology
- Cognitive impairment
- Psychiatric illness
- Diabetes

CASE STUDY: ELIZABETH TAYLOR

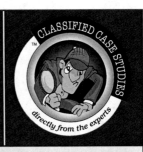

Elizabeth Taylor will be remembered for many reasons, ranging from her famous roles in movies such as *Cleopatra* and *Cat on a Hot Tin Roof* to her eight marriages to her co-founding the American Foundation for AIDS Research. Despite her beauty and her fame, age and injuries caused her many years of ill health before she died from congestive heart failure at age 79 in 2011.

Taylor, who was born with scoliosis, was thrown from a horse at the age of 12 while filming *National Velvet*; she sustained a spinal fracture and underwent multiple back surgeries and drug rehab stays as a result. By age 78, she had undergone a total of five back surgeries and more than 100 operations in all. Collectively, these procedures along with continued weight gain took a toll on her body and she was eventually confined to a wheelchair.

Taylor essentially lived her whole life with severe back pain. She had discs removed and replaced with bones from other parts of her body. Some of her health issues were likely unrelated to her scoliosis and back issues, but there is no doubt most of them tied in with those chronic issues and her attempt to work in spite of them. At the end of her life, she was reportedly practically bedridden and "too tired and weak" to undergo additional surgeries.

In addition to the musculoskeletal system, other systems are affected. Atherosclerosis (a disease in which plaque builds up in the arteries) and cardiovascular disease may result from physical inactivity. Prolonged bed rest can increase the risk of blood clots forming, resulting in pulmonary embolism. Without activity the lungs do not exercise. The resulting reduction in muscle strength and endurance causes less movement of the diaphragm, intercostal and abdominal muscles. This leads to secretions pooling, a cough and the development of pneumonia. Weight-bearing intolerance can also affect the gastrointestinal track and cause decreased appetite, lower gastric secretions, constipation, impaired absorption and atrophy of the gastrointestinal tract cell linings. Kidney stones and urinary tract infections develop as a result of increased excretion of water and salt. Cognition is also affected; some people have difficulty with focusing, judgment and problem solving. A whole host of psychiatric illnesses can develop centered upon anxiety, fear and depression. Glucose intolerance develops along with other metabolic alterations such as changes in temperature, sweating and circadian rhythm.

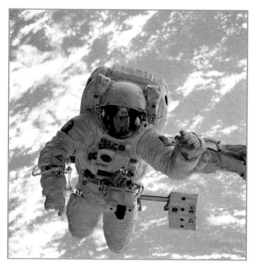

The medical conditions that occur with weight-bearing intolerance are similar to those that occur to astronauts working in microgravity. NASA has studied this subject extensively since it was founded in 1958. Astronauts who work in space perform physically demanding work in a challenging environment. They have been found to have an increased risk for musculoskeletal injury. It has also been noticed that there is a threefold higher injury rate during mission periods then outside of mission periods. Living in space causes the astronauts' body to change. On earth, we carry our weight on our lower body or legs. This weight bearing keeps them strong. In space, astronauts float freely. They begin to lose strength in their legs, back and bones. So how do astronauts overcome this development? They exercise every day. In space their heart and blood undergo changes as well. When we stand on earth the blood goes to our legs. But in space astronauts do not stand, so the heart has to work extra hard to move blood from the upper body and brain where it tends to pool to the lower body. The brain thinks there is too much blood there so it enters a protective state and tells the body to make less bloods, which results in the body dehydrating itself. This eventually weakens the astronaut to the point of fainting.

Stroke, Brain Insults and Other Neurologic Conditions

Stroke

A cerebrovascular accident is the proper medical term for a stroke. A stroke is the interruption of blood flow to your brain. A stroke may occur as a result of a blockage or a rupture of a blood vessel. There are important signs and symptoms to be aware of and the timing of diagnosis is absolutely critical. The faster a suspected stroke reaches medical attention, the more quickly it is treated and the better the prognosis. Undiagnosed stroke or the delayed treatment of a stroke may result in permanent brain damage.

An ischemic stroke occurs when a blood vessel going to the brain is blocked. The rupture of a blood vessel in the brain is what is referred to as a hemorrhagic stroke. This prevents blood from getting to that part of the brain, and when the brain is deprived of blood and oxygen it causes the brain cells to die. In an embolic stroke, a blood clot may form in a remote area and get lodged in the brain's blood vessels.

The signs and symptoms of a stroke are:

- Sudden headache
- Nausea, vomiting, or dizziness
- Difficulty walking

- Loss of balance
- Loss of coordination
- Difficulty speaking
- Difficulty understanding those speaking
- Numbness or paralysis of the face, arm, leg or side of the body
- Blurred or diminished vision

These signs and symptoms may occur suddenly and continue to worsen with time. It is very important to see a physician immediately for a history and physical examination. Various tests such as a blood test, an MRI scan, CT scan, angiogram and/or carotid ultrasound may need to be performed.

The treatment of a stroke is dependent upon the type. In an **ischemic stroke** the blockage needs to be removed or opened. Oftentimes this is performed by a clot dissolving drug or blood thinner. Occasionally surgery does need to be performed. With a **hemorrhagic stroke** the treatment is directed towards controlling bleeding and removing blood clots that may be putting pressure on the brain. The treatment for hemorrhagic stroke may either be a drug that lowers the pressure in your brain caused by the bleeding or surgery to remove blood clots and/or repair ruptured vessels.

After a stroke the recovery period is dependent upon how severe the stroke was. Rehabilitation is often needed. Rehabilitation services may include speech therapy, occupational therapy and physical therapy.

Obesity, an unhealthy diet and too little exercise are associated with increased risk of stroke. The risk in obese men and women compared to leaner men and women is at least twice as much. It is estimated that 80 percent of all strokes are preventable. In order to prevent a stroke, risk factors need to be addressed.

PREVENTION

One should prevent heart and cardiovascular disease by:

- Exercising regularly
- Maintaining a diet rich in fruits and vegetables
- Maintaining a healthy weight
- Controlling diabetes
- Stopping smoking
- Using alcohol in moderation
- Maintaining a normal blood pressure
- Limiting saturated fats and cholesterol

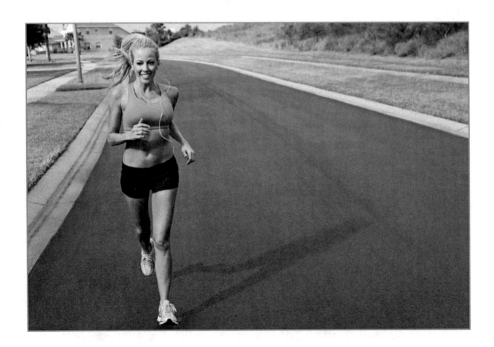

If you are a known risk for stroke, drugs that thin the blood and prevent clot formation may be needed. The recovery from a stroke may take weeks, months or years. The prognosis and speed of recovery are dependent upon which area of the brain is affected and the length of time it was affected.

Head injuries

Head injuries are any form of injury to the brain, skull or scalp. Injuries may vary from mild to severe, they may be closed or open, and there may be a concussion or scalp wound involved. Head injury may occur from trauma such as a gunshot, motor vehicle accident, fall on your head, assault or violent shaking injury.

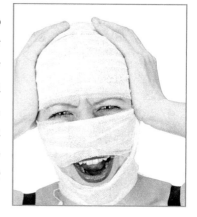

The symptoms of a head injury are dependent upon the type of head injury. Mild head injury symptoms include ringing in the year, temporary memory loss, nausea, headache, confusion, inability to stand and/or small cuts or bumps. Severe head injury symptoms include bleeding from a cut or scalp wound, loss of consciousness, loss of muscle control, seizures, vomiting, inability to focus the eyes and abnormal eye movements. Mild symptoms may become severe with time.

The diagnosis of a head injury is made based on history and physical examination, X-rays, CT scan and/or MRI scan. A head injury requires emergency evaluation and care. Emergency medical technicians should stabilize the victim prior to transporting him or her to the hospital.

Head injuries may be treated by either medications to control blood clotting or seizures or surgery to stop bleeding in the brain and reduce brain swelling. If observation is recommended, careful monitoring of the level of consciousness is necessary.

The outcome of a head injury depends upon the severity of the injury and the length of time it takes to diagnose and treat that injury. Lifelong changes to the level of consciousness, personality or behavior, and physical abilities such as walking, talking, dressing and eating may occur. Alternatively, symptoms may resolve with time and further medical treatment. Head injury prevention should focus on the wearing of helmets when riding bicycles or motorcycles, and avoidance of headfirst diving.

CASE STUDY: FRANKLIN ROOSEVELT

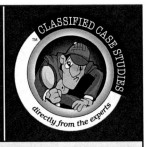

Despite extreme efforts to hide his maladies while he was in office, it is now widely known that President Franklin D. Roosevelt suffered from a significant physical disability. In 1921, when Roosevelt was vacationing, he manifested symptoms of polio or — as it was commonly known then — infantile paralysis. In hindsight, some physicians believe that Roosevelt's paralytic illness was actually Guillain-Barré syndrome. Nevertheless Roosevelt developed total and permanent paralysis from the waist down and had to use a wheelchair thereafter.

Roosevelt spent some time in rehabilitation efforts where he attempted for several years to recover from his paralysis. He began swimming three times a week, which allowed him to strengthen his arms, stomach and lower back while achieving normal function in his nervous system. As a result, he was fitted with braces in 1922 that locked at the knee and continued the length of this leg; these allowed him to stand with assistance and eventually enabled him to walk on his own. These braces were key in his efforts to never appear in a wheelchair in public.

Roosevelt was reportedly very positive in his attitude regarding his disability. While he took strong measures to not be perceived as "weak" in the public eye, he also did not allow his disability to depress him or create limitations. He visited hot springs as a method of treatment and rejuvenation and continued to maintain his heath in every way to make it easier for him to live with his disability.

Paraplegia and Quadriplegia

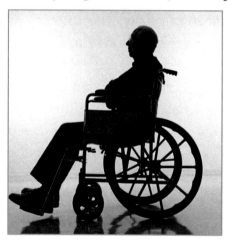 The most common association with wheelchairs is paralysis. There are many causes of paralysis, but the results are all the same. **Paraplegia** is a paralysis that involves the lower extremities. **Quadriplegia** involves both the upper and lower extremities. Most people with paraplegia and quadriplegia are wheelchair dependent at least initially, and must continue to use a wheelchair if recovery does not occur. Paraplegia is the most common form of paralysis, while quadriplegia accounts for one third of all spinal cord injuries.

The signs and symptoms of damage to the spinal cord include:

- Motor disorders (weakness of muscles)
- Pain
- Sensory abnormalities
- Bowel and bladder disorders
- Genital and sexual disorders
- Breathing problems

- Autonomic nervous system abnormalities
- Other systems involvement (i.e. skin, skeleton, etc.)

The motor system disorders involved with injury include voluntary and involuntary (autonomic motor control) motor systems. The voluntary motor control involves the muscles that move the arms and legs. Damage to those muscles may result in complete (no movement possible) or incomplete (movement is possible but weak) paralysis. The involuntary or autonomic motor system regulates the tone of muscle and injury can either result in hypertonia/spasticity (high resistance to passive movement), or hypotonia/flaccid paralysis (low resistance to movement). Sensory disorders resulting from paralysis include superficial sensibility and deep sensibility. Superficial sensibility loss involves the complete lack (anesthesia) or partial loss (hypoesthesia) of the senses of touch, pain, temperature and gross feeling. Deep sensibility loss results in the anesthesia or hypoesthesia of the ability to determine the position of the body in space.

Bowel and bladder abnormalities are due to nerve damage to those organ systems that have affected the motor and sensory nerves resulting in changes of reflexes. Depending upon which nerves are affected, different injury patterns and management will have to be considered.

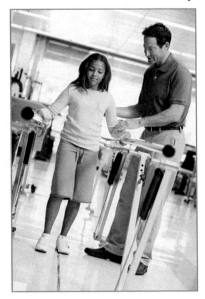

Involvement of the neck and upper back can result in autonomic disorders. There may be autonomic dysreflexia (an uncontrolled elevation of the blood pressure), body temperature variations, or pain that is difficult to control.

Genital and sexual disorders involving both men and women may result from spinal cord injury. Men may be unable to achieve erections or ejaculation, while women may develop analgesia of the perineum area, resulting in difficulty achieving orgasm and challenges during labor.

Spinal injury may also affect the respiratory muscles. The abdominal, intercostal and diaphragm muscles control breathing. When there is involvement of the nerves that innervate those muscles then various respiratory disorders occur, ranging from breathing to simple coughing.

Lastly various other disorders in other systems may occur ranging from cardiovascular to bone demineralization. Paralysis touches on every system in the body. Some systems are affected more than others but rarely are any spared.

PRIORITIZATION OF TREATMENT

The prioritization of treatment for those with paralysis is:

- Initial treatment — resuscitation and surgery
- Rehabilitation
- Physical therapy
- Occupational therapy
- Recreational activities including sports
- Bowel and bladder retraining exercises
- Prevention of pressure sores
- Preparation for returning home

The evaluation and treatment of paralysis is extremely complicated. We should focus on the prevention of acute traumatic injuries to decrease the number of wheelchair dependents. Regarding the cervical spine, injury can be decreased by the Feet First – First Time program to decrease diving injuries. Regarding the thoracic and lumbar spine, injuries may be decreased by always wearing a seatbelt while in the car.

CASE STUDY: CHRISTOPHER REEVE

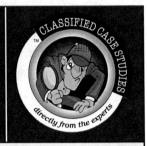

Christopher Reeve was an American actor best known for his portrayal of Superman in four films and for his struggle to live and thrive as a quadriplegic years later. In 1995, at age 42, Reeve broke his neck during an equestrian competition and was left paralyzed and unable to breathe without the help of a respirator. He suffered fractures to his top two vertebrae and damaged his spinal cord.

Despite the severity of his injury, Reeve neither ended his career nor ceased to be active in causes he believed in. In 1997, he made his directorial debut with *In the Gloaming* on HBO, which was met with rave reviews. He published an autobiography titled *Still Me* in 1998. In 1999, he appeared in a remake of Hitchcock's thriller *Rear Window*.

While not everyone has the resources and opportunities that Reeve did after his injury, great strives have been made to open doors for paralyzed individuals. Reeve has been a driving force behind much of these improvements. He served as Chairman of the Board of a nonprofit organization that supported research that developed treatments for paralysis caused by spinal cord injuries and central nervous system disorders. His greatest achievements include helping pass landmark legislation and raising awareness about the importance of the challenges facing those with disabilities.

Reeve died at the age of 52 from a cardiac arrest caused by systemic infection.

Spinal Stenosis

Spinal stenosis is the narrowing of the canal that contains the spinal cord and spinal nerves. The purpose of the spinal canal is to protect these sensitive nerves. The bony structures of the spinal cord form a ring around the spinal cord and nerve roots. There are many causes of spinal stenosis. Some people are born with a too-small spinal canal, resulting in early pressure on the spinal cord or nerve roots. Others develop the narrowing due to pressure from arthritis, bone fracture, tumor or infection, which all place pressure on the neural structures. Yet the most common cause of spinal stenosis is aging. With aging the body tends to shrink as a result of a wearing out of the discs. This loss of height, coupled with the infolding of tough ligaments from years of wear and tear as well as bone spurs or arthritis developing on the bones, adds additional circumferential pressure on the spinal cord or nerves. This pressure causes space in the spine to narrow. The most common (75 percent of cases) location for spinal stenosis is in the low back or lumbar spine.

A pinching of the spinal cord or nerves can result from spinal stenosis. This compression on the neural structures may result in a loss of muscle power or weakness and/or abnormal feelings in the arms or legs such as numbness or tingling. This compression of the nerves may result in difficulty using your arms or hands, pain in the arms or legs, difficulty walking, frequent falling, clumsiness, numbness and tingling, or hot and cold feelings in the arms and legs. As symptoms continue to worsen, people with spinal stenosis gradually lose their ability to move on their own and develop a more sedentary lifestyle. **With the development of a more sedentary lifestyle a whole host of body functions begin to deteriorate — muscle atrophies, fat builds, bones begin to soften and thinking starts to cloud.** This inactivity also results in a higher incidence of diabetes, hypertension, heart disease and cancer. This process becomes compounding with time.

The treatment of early spinal stenosis includes postural changes and nonsteroidal anti-inflammatory medications. Should symptoms continue, a diagnostic study such as an MRI may be performed to give an accurate diagnosis.

Treatment of spinal stenosis ranges from activity modification to postural change to weight loss to nonsteroidal anti-inflammatories to physical therapy to low-level laser therapy to injections with steroids or other numbing medications to surgery.

Remember that spinal stenosis is a structural problem and that inactivity due to spinal stenosis can become a death march for seniors. In order for seniors to remain independent they must stay active. How healthy a senior is is reflected directly in how fast and how long he or she can walk. The inability to walk a distance is an early sign of a senior who is in the process of losing his or her independence and will eventually require a mobility aid such as a cane, walker or wheelchair to move safely from one point to another. Remember the longer you wait through various nonoperative treatment plans, the more the senior's vitality deteriorates, and the higher surgical risks become.

If you develop a neurologic deficit or paralysis, or have severe incapacitating pain that interferes with the quality of your life that does not improve with nonoperative care for the treatment of spinal stenosis, surgery may be considered. The main goal in surgery is to remove the structure that is compressing the spinal cord or nerve. This form of decompression surgery may be performed in the low back by laminectomy, laminotomy, foraminotomy and/or discectomy. In the neck this surgery may be performed either from the back of the neck by a laminectomy or laminotomy, or from the front of the neck by a discectomy and reconstructive procedure (fusion and internal fixation). More recently less invasive procedures have become available. Those less invasive procedures for the low back often employ interspinous devices coupled with microdecompressions.

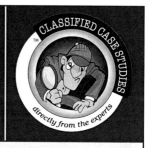

CASE STUDY:
SAMUEL L. JACKSON

An actor known for a wide-range of roles, Samuel Jackson's movies include *Shaft*, *Pulp Fiction*, and the *Star Wars* prequels. While filming *S.W.A.T.*, Jackson says he woke up one morning and could not move. He rolled out of bed, crawled to the bathroom, took some Advil, and eventually ended up getting an epidural steroid injection so he could finish the movie. When it wrapped, he had to have a cyst removed from his sciatic nerve.

To achieve a pain-free status, he reports undergoing regular acupuncture sessions (twice per week) and having a titanium bolt put in his spine, which was fitted to allow him to walk, bend over and even play golf.

In 2012, the FDA approved the Coflex® Interlaminar Stabilization ™ device (Paradigm Spine, New York, New York). The device offers motion preserving, non-fusion stabilization after a surgical decompression for moderate-to-sever spinal stenosis. Jackson appeared on *The Ellen Show* in 2015 to relate his experience with the device and how it has helped relieve his back issues.

The outlook for surgery is dependent upon the severity and duration of the symptoms at the time of initial treatment, the individual's response to treatment, the underlying medical conditions of the patient, and how neglected their disease process has become. National Institute of Arthritis and Musculoskeletal and Skin Diseases (NIAMS) supported researchers have published results from the Spine Patient Outcomes Research Trial (SPORT), the largest trial today comparing surgical and nonsurgical treatments for low back pain and sciatica caused by spinal stenosis. The study found that patients with spinal stenosis were most effectively treated by surgery for relief of symptoms and improving function. Although the functional status of the patients who received nonoperative treatment still improved, it lagged behind the improvement for the surgical patient group. Yet one must remember that all surgery carries risks, and those surgeries that involve general anesthesia and older patients have potential for additional risks and complications. The most common complication after surgery is durotomy, or a tear of the surrounding membrane of the spinal cord. Other potential complications include infection, blood clots either in the extremities or at the surgical site, or other medical conditions and comorbidities. One must remember that the healthier you are at the time of the surgical procedure directly correlates with the percentage of complications that may occur.

Obesity and Morbid Obesity

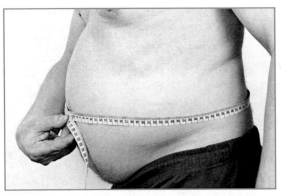

Obesity is a condition where one has too much weight on their body frame. In this condition one has a high body mass index (BMI), or too much weight for their height. Being overweight may be caused by your bone structure, high bone density, or excess body fat. Morbid obesity occurs when the excess body fat begins to endanger your overall health.

Every person requires a certain number of calories per day, which is converted into energy for your body to use. The body makes that energy run your muscles and vital organs. Any calories that are not used for energy conversion become converted into body fat. So eating more calories per day than what your body requires results in the development of excess fat. Daily activity level also plays a role in burning off those calories. Inactivity results in weight gain. Weight gain may also come as a result of medications, medical diseases such as hypothyroidism, genetic factors, hormonal changes related to pregnancy or menopause, and is often a psychological result of stress and anxiety. Anyone can gain weight and become obese if they allow themselves more calories than their body can use.

Body Mass Index Table

	Normal						Overweight					Obese										Extreme Obesity														
BMI	19	20	21	22	23	24	25	26	27	28	29	30	31	32	33	34	35	36	37	38	39	40	41	42	43	44	45	46	47	48	49	50	51	52	53	54
Height (inches)												Body Weight (pounds)																								
58	91	96	100	105	110	115	119	124	129	134	138	143	148	153	158	162	167	172	177	181	186	191	196	201	205	210	215	220	224	229	234	239	244	248	253	258
59	94	99	104	109	114	119	124	128	133	138	143	148	153	158	163	168	173	178	183	188	193	198	203	208	212	217	222	227	232	237	242	247	252	257	262	267
60	97	102	107	112	118	123	128	133	138	143	148	153	158	163	168	174	179	184	189	194	199	204	209	215	220	225	230	235	240	245	250	255	261	266	271	276
61	100	106	111	116	122	127	132	137	143	148	153	158	164	169	174	180	185	190	195	201	206	211	217	222	227	232	238	243	248	254	259	264	269	275	280	285
62	104	109	115	120	126	131	136	142	147	153	158	164	169	175	180	186	191	196	202	207	213	218	224	229	235	240	246	251	256	262	267	273	278	284	289	295
63	107	113	118	124	130	135	141	146	152	158	163	169	175	180	186	191	197	203	208	214	220	225	231	237	242	248	254	259	265	270	278	282	287	293	299	304
64	110	116	122	128	134	140	145	151	157	163	169	174	180	186	192	197	204	209	215	221	227	232	238	244	250	256	262	267	273	279	285	291	296	302	308	314
65	114	120	126	132	138	144	150	156	162	168	174	180	186	192	198	204	210	216	222	228	234	240	246	252	258	264	270	276	282	288	294	300	306	312	318	324
66	118	124	130	136	142	148	155	161	167	173	179	186	192	198	204	210	216	223	229	235	241	247	253	260	266	272	278	284	291	297	303	309	315	322	328	334
67	121	127	134	140	146	153	159	166	172	178	185	191	198	204	211	217	223	230	236	242	249	255	261	268	274	280	287	293	299	306	312	319	325	331	338	344
68	125	131	138	144	151	158	164	171	177	184	190	197	203	210	216	223	230	236	243	249	256	262	269	276	282	289	295	302	308	315	322	328	335	341	348	354
69	128	135	142	149	155	162	169	176	182	189	196	203	209	216	223	230	236	243	250	257	263	270	277	284	291	297	304	311	318	324	331	338	345	351	358	365
70	132	139	146	153	160	167	174	181	188	195	202	209	216	222	229	236	243	250	257	264	271	278	285	292	299	306	313	320	327	334	341	348	355	362	369	376
71	136	143	150	157	165	172	179	186	193	200	208	215	222	229	236	243	250	257	265	272	279	286	293	301	308	315	322	329	338	343	351	358	365	372	379	386
72	140	147	154	162	169	177	184	191	199	206	213	221	228	235	242	250	258	265	272	279	287	294	302	309	316	324	331	338	346	353	361	368	375	383	390	397
73	144	151	159	166	174	182	189	197	204	212	219	227	235	242	250	257	265	272	280	288	295	302	310	318	325	333	340	348	355	363	371	378	386	393	401	408
74	148	155	163	171	179	186	194	202	210	218	225	233	241	249	256	264	272	280	287	295	303	311	319	326	334	342	350	358	365	373	381	389	396	404	412	420
75	152	160	168	176	184	192	200	208	216	224	232	240	248	256	264	272	279	287	295	303	311	319	327	335	343	351	359	367	375	383	391	399	407	415	423	431
76	156	164	172	180	189	197	205	213	221	230	238	246	254	263	271	279	287	295	304	312	320	328	336	344	353	361	369	377	385	394	402	410	418	426	435	443

Source: Adapted from Clinical Guidelines on the Identification, Evaluation, and Treatment of Overweight and Obesity in Adults: The Evidence Report.

Obesity is defined as a BMI greater than 30. BMI is calculated as an estimate of your body fat using your height and weight. Visit **www.bmi-calculator.net** to calculate your BMI. Obesity can result in serious health problems such as heart disease, osteoarthritis, stroke, sleep apnea and diabetes. It is estimated that the morbidly obese have a six times higher incidence of developing heart disease as compared to people of normal health. A BMI between 18.5 and 24.9 is generally considered normal. A person who is 100 pounds (BMI of 40 or greater) above their ideal body weight is considered to be morbidly obese.

The traditional treatment for obesity is diet and exercise. If these methods prove unsuccessful and weight loss is necessary due to the risk of diabetes, heart disease and sleep apnea — which are associated with severe obesity — then consider laparoscopic banding, laparoscopic gastric sleeve or gastric bypass surgery. Consulting a bariatric surgeon is important to understand the pros and cons of each surgical procedure.

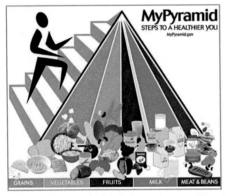

Rather than waiting to become morbidly obese and develop the associated serious and potentially life threatening conditions, be proactive and start treatment today. To diet successfully you should eat more fruits and vegetables, partake in smaller meals, count calories and avoid highly processed foods that are high in fat and sugar. The addition of a daily exercise program is important to increase your heart rate and sweat on a daily basis. You should try walking, jogging, swimming, biking or some other activity that requires exertion. Just think of the astronauts' daily exercise requirements.

There are many prescription weight loss and appetite suppressant drugs. Doctors may prescribe them if your BMI is 30 or higher. There are many prescription weight loss drugs available. All these drugs have specific uses and a host of side effects and/or complications. Your physician needs to carefully monitor you to prevent any unwanted results.

CASE STUDY: MANUEL URIBE AND DEREK MITCHELL

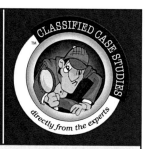

At times, individuals end up with severe back pain and become wheelchair bound simply because they allowed themselves to become morbidly obese. At some point, the body's joints become unable to support the weight being carried and walking becomes uncomfortable. When that happens, the person begins an ugly cycle where their inactivity leads to continued weight gain and the extra weight leads to greater inactivity.

Manuel Uribe was at one time the world's heaviest man (as defined by the Guinness Book of Records), weighing 1,230 pounds. At that weight, he was not even able to enjoy the benefits of a wheelchair, but instead had not left his bed for six years. In 2014, he died at the age of 48, after suffering from liver and cardiac conditions.

Uribe led a sedentary life, with a sedentary job as a repair technician. He said he never exercised and ate a normal Mexican diet of beans, rice, flour tortilla, corn tortilla, French fries, hamburgers, subs and pizzas. He was already trending toward obesity when his divorce led to depression and greater weight gain. He got into his bed and never got out.

His physical cause of death was not surprising, but his life also highlights the negative impact clinical depression and other mental health disorders can have on individual's physical well being. It is important that if a person is suffering from emotional or psychological issues that could led to inactivity that they seek medical help for all issues contributing to their weight problems.

Derek Mitchell, on the other hand, was able to realize that, when he reached 625 pounds, he needed to set fitness goals for himself that would prevent him from ending up in a wheelchair or worse fate. One of these goals, he completed in March of 2015 (at 570 pounds) when he finished the Big 12 Run in Kansas City, Missouri where he lives. The race stretches just past three miles.

At the start of 2015, Mitchell made the commitment to cut soda from his diet, eat healthier and go on daily walks. That got him started on his weight loss path, but it was his sister, a marathon runner, who suggested he make it a goal to attempt a 5K. He agreed not only to just complete one, but to complete one per month for the year.

"As soon as I saw that finish line and heard everybody yelling, all the pain that I'd been feeling up until that point vanished," Mitchell reported to *Runner's World* magazine. He completed that 5K in 1:27:44 and is striving to trim time off every 5K he completes thereafter.

More than five years before this marathon journey began, Mitchell was diagnosed with a non-cancerous brain tumor on his pituitary gland that prevents his body from producing testosterone. Among other things, testosterone controls metabolism, energy and drive — making it far too easy to gain weight and much more difficult to lose it.

However, Mitchell's commitment in 2015 was undeniable and he more than fulfilled his goal of completing one 5K per month. In fact, he earned medals and bibs from 20 5Ks and two 10Ks while dropping about 100 pounds. He is undoubtedly healthier and committed to racing more, running more and dropping more weight. All of his efforts should keep him moving and prevent him following a similar path to that of Manuel Uribe.

Osteoarthritis

Osteoarthritis (OA) is known as degenerative joint disease or the "wear and tear" arthritis of aging. In OA the cartilage (the cushion between the joints) breaks down, resulting in pain, swelling and/or stiffness. Twenty seven million Americans are affected. It is most common in people over 65. Risk factors include increased age, obesity, overuse or abuse of a joint, weak musculature and genetic factors.

After the breakdown of cartilage occurs, bones also begin to deteriorate and form bone spurs. The fragments of bone or cartilage may break off and initiate an inflammatory response that further damages the joint. This damage to the joint eventually leads to complete joint destruction and pain.

Symptoms include:

- Joint warmth
- Swelling
- Pain
- Clicking or cracking sounds
- Stiffness or limited range of motion

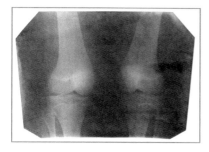 Osteoarthritis may affect different parts of the body including the hips, knees, fingers, feet and spine. A diagnosis of osteoarthritis is usually made by joint aspiration, X-ray, or MRI scan.

Treatment includes:

- Strengthening exercises
- Weight management
- Stretching
- Pain and anti-inflammatory medications
- Surgery

Previously we believed that osteoarthritis was a result of the wear and tear of joint cartilage. Cartilage is the white and slightly elastic substance that covers the ends of our bones and allows them to slide against each other. However, the real problem seems to be in the cartilage cells called chondrocytes. For a chondrocyte to be healthy, it is important for it to receive oxygen and nutrients so that cartilage regeneration can continue. Chondrocytes also hate violent blows, as they develop an inflammatory reaction that becomes extremely painful. In order to oxygenate and nourish your chondrocytes, it is important that the synovial fluid in a joint be allowed to move around and feed and oxygenate your chondrocytes. To do this you must keep your joints moving through low level exercises such as walking, yoga and tai chi. Also, carrying too much weight puts added pressure on the joints.

Inflammation may be controlled by a diet rich in antioxidants, so try eating more fresh fruits and vegetables. Add spices that have an anti-inflammatory property such as cloves, red pepper, turmeric, cinnamon, ginger or rosemary to your food. Try incorporating more dark, leafy vegetables such as spinach, kale and collard greens into your diet. Garlic, onions, berries, green tea and omega-3s also seem to help. Avoidance of injury and maintaining healthy chondrocytes are the best ways to prevent, delay or improve the symptoms of osteoarthritis.

CASE STUDY: GEORGE H. W. BUSH

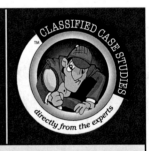

President George H.W. Bush suffered from medical issues that restricted his ability to walk in 2012; these issues stemmed from Vascular Parkinsonism and a hip replacement. Bush was interviewed in Parade magazine that year and explained that the disease "just affects the legs." "It's not painful," he explained. "You tell your legs to move, and they don't. It's strange, but if you have to have some bad-sounding disease, this is a good one to get."

Bush had been an active person prior to the onset of this disease, and had been limited to using a scooter or wheelchair as a result. Still, the former Navy pilot refused to let a little thing like limited mobility slow him down. In 2014, Bush celebrated his 90th birthday by skydiving out of a helicopter (with a tandem skydiver) near his summer home in Maine. Prior to his disease, he had celebrated his 75th, 80th, and 85th birthdays the same way and decided not to break the tradition.

In 2015, Bush was hospitalized after a fall where he broke his C2 vertebrae in his neck. Doctors who treated him reported that there were no resulting neurological issues despite the severity of the injury itself. After his stay in the hospital, he was set to be fitted for a brace and receive physical therapy. At 91, he was expected to heal more slowly, but still to make a full recovery.

As it turns out, just a few months later, despite being in a wheelchair and wearing a neck brace, Bush still rolled onto the baseball diamond of a Houston Astros game and threw out the first pitch of the game.

Commonality of the Causes

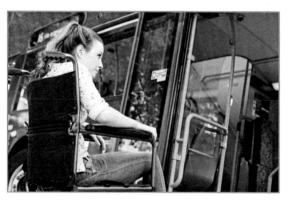

There are many causes of wheelchair use. Paralysis from neurologic origin still remains high on the list. Paralysis may be described as a loss of movement or function. It is caused by damage to the nervous system — either central or peripheral. It may be temporary or permanent. Temporary paralysis occurs during sleep or during the use of drugs such as curare. Permanent paralysis may be caused by trauma, either bacterial or viral infection, metabolic issues such as diabetes or exposure to heavy metals, a tumor, or another indeterminate cause. People may also be born with permanent paralysis, such as those with cerebral palsy.

Whether the central or peripheral nervous system is involved, or the patient is young or old, length of time compression of neural tissue is important for predicting reversibility. The speed of recovery is an important feature. The prognosis is generally determined in the first weeks after the onset of paralysis. After two months with no sign of recovery, the recovery potential decreases very quickly over time. However, no definite conclusion can be drawn until at least eight months after onset of spinal cord symptoms and 18 months after onset of nerve root or peripheral nerve symptoms.

In order to determine the cause of a neurologic deficit or a painful condition, you first need an accurate diagnosis. A careful history and physical examination by a skilled physician is the first step. A tentative diagnosis can be obtained at this time. The diagnosis obtains objective information via radiologic imaging. Imaging may take the form of X-rays, CT scan, MRI scan, myelogram with follow-up CT scan and/or discography. Electrodiagnostic studies via electromyography study (EMG), somatosensory evoked potentials (SSEP), and motor evoked potentials (MEP) will give information regarding neurologic dysfunction. Finally, needle or open biopsy may be needed for confirmation of an offending organism or pathologic condition such as cancer.

With the epidemic rise of obesity in this country, the development of inactivity, osteoarthritis and multiple comorbidities are reaching crisis levels regarding health care consumption. The cycle begins with musculoskeletal joint pain that limits activities at work and home, resulting in decreased mobility, decreased physical activities and ultimately weight gain. Weight gain causes joint pressure and pain to increase, which results in osteoarthritis. With the combination of obesity and inactivity, a whole host of metabolic diseases develop including hypertension, heart disease, diabetes, cancer and depression. The key to breaking the cycle is movement. Wheelchair use is made worse by the disease of inactivity.

My coach used to say "Boys, either use it or lose it," and I never really understood what he was trying to say. Over time I have come to understand the following facts:

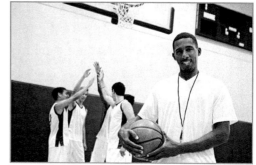

1. Inactivity results in the loss of muscle strength in both older and younger people and increases with age.

2. A young person who does not use their legs for two weeks will lose one third of their muscle strength, while older people will lose one fourth of their muscle strength.

3. Older people have less muscle mass than younger people.

4. Inactive people have less muscle mass than active people.

5. Women are more likely to be sedentary than men.

6. Non-Hispanic white males are more likely to engage in physical activity than Hispanic or non-Hispanic black males.

7. The more muscle you have, the more muscle you lose after injury.

8. After injury, the loss of muscle mass in older or inactive people has a greater impact on their general health and quality of life.

9. After muscle mass loss, you can multiply the period of loss by three to determine the amount of time it will take to recover.

10. Cycling or walking will help you regain lost muscle mass, but if you want to regain your muscular strength following a period of inactivity, weight training is essential.

Because of these facts, it is essential that inactivity is minimized after surgery and rehabilitation begins as soon as possible. If you want to eventually recover all of your pre-surgery abilities, prolonged activity must be avoided. For those who choose or are forced into a sedentary lifestyle, the chance of wheelchair use preceding death significantly increases.

Less active, less fit people have a greater risk of developing:

- Hypertension
- Heart disease
- Anxiety and depression
- Cancer
- Diabetes
- High cholesterol

It should also be recognized that patients with chronic disease, paralysis and cancer are also subjected to the same risks as those who elect to be inactive. With this disease of inactivity, weight may either decrease or increase depending upon the presence of a chronic disease. Those with chronic diseases often develop **wasting syndrome**, which results in a weight decrease, whereas those sedentary individuals without a disease usually gain significant amounts of weight, worsening their already precarious situation.

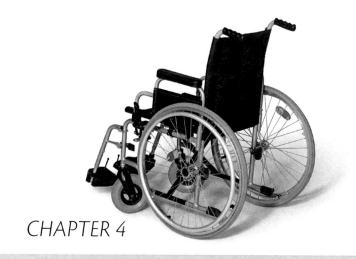

CHAPTER 4

AVOIDING THE CHAIR

There is a specific group of people that is going to spend the rest of their lives in a wheelchair due to an injury or disease. There is another group of people that were forced into a wheelchair after sustaining an injury or developing a disease, but still have the potential to recover. And lastly there is a group of people with self-inflicted diseases that will eventually force them into a wheelchair. If you are in this last group, just think of what it will be like to wear a diaper, be dependent on a wheelchair, and have to ask your friends or family to help you with activities of daily living.

People become wheelchair dependent for many different reasons. It is important to realize when you head down a specific path it is often hard to change directions. But sometimes you get lucky and get a second chance. Through hard work, dedication, perseverance and retraining, the path can be altered.

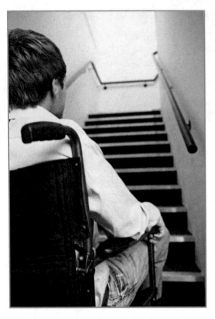

How does one go about changing the path? First it is important to have a positive attitude. Following attitude, nutrition and exercise are also important to reverse the cycle of wheelchair dependency. Remember that exercise includes both physical and mental programs.

For those who are not yet wheelchair dependent, taking better care of yourself now may pay off in the future, just like a small seed planted now may one day grow into a healthy tree. By preventing self-inflicted disease, you can help prevent limited mobility and wheelchair dependence.

Activities of daily living (ADLs) are the things we would normally do during the course of the day. Daily living activities generally include self-care activities such as feeding ourselves, dressing, grooming, bathing/showering, and homemaking as well as leisure activities. The ability or inability to perform these activities of daily living is a measure of your level of ability or impairment.

If you develop a minor neurologic deficit, the impairment may be limited. If you develop a major neurologic deficit (quadriplegia/paraplegia), then there will be significant challenges to your activities of daily living. In the case that you become impaired, you will have to consider how you will accomplish each of the activities of daily living listed above. The goal is independence.

Avoiding Re-injury or Relapse

In order to recover from an injury or illness there are three action steps you should take.

KEY ELEMENTS FOR HEALING

The three key elements for healing yourself after an injury or illness are:

1. Use good pain science data
2. Remember that sometimes less is more
3. Have a carefully constructed rehabilitation program

Paying attention to these three elements helps prevent re-injury and allows for a steady, progressive recovery.

Think of a child on a family road trip. Every 10 minutes the child asks, "When are we going to get there?" The more he asks, the faster he wants to get there, and the longer the trip seems to take. The same is true for recovery from an injury or illness.

RECOVERY FACTORS

Recovery is dependent upon a multitude of factors:

1. Magnitude of injury/ pathology
2. Length of time of compression of structures
3. Age
4. Comorbidities or other medical conditions
5. Substance issues (alcohol, tobacco and illicit drugs)
6. When treatment was received

Keeping Active

Trying to maintain a physical activity level? Trying to lose weight? Ever think about getting some objective data? Recently physical activity monitors have been introduced. The activity monitor is a small flexible band that fits on your wrist. It syncs with your computer/smartphone and works like a pedometer, but better. The objective is to take 10,000 steps/day, which translates into approximately 4 miles. When the person

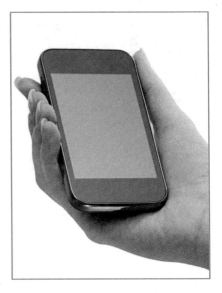

reaches 10,000 steps the device vibrates. By syncing it with your smartphone/computer you can monitor your progress every week. You can also track calories and sleep hours if you wish.

Remember that this is only a device that tracks activity level. It is a start. It can also be a motivational tool to do better than you did the day before. Try it. You may like it, and it may motivate you. But for the wheelchair dependent, the monitor needs to be modified into one that tracks upper extremity movement.

Avoiding Accidents

Most accidents happen at home. We spend most of our time at home but think little about our safety. Many falls can be prevented by making simple changes.

How to fall-proof your home:

- Improve lighting
- Install handrails and grab bars

- Make items more easily reachable
- Remove anything that you could trip on
- Give plenty of walking room by arranging furniture
- Remove throw rugs and secure carpeting
- Place nonslip strips on floors and steps
- Clean spills immediately
- Be careful walking on outdoor steps
- Take ice precautions
- Improve lighting
- Place grab bars in your tub or shower

Falling is the number one cause for fracture. Falling and sustaining a hip or spinal fracture often results in higher mortality risk for seniors. There may also be a physical reason for your falls, like spinal stenosis.

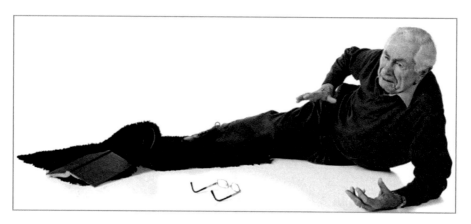

Avoiding Whiplash

A car's headrest is not designed to rest your head against it and relax while driving. The headrest is designed to prevent a whiplash injury in a rear-end collision. Motor vehicles purchased within the last five years have literally become a pain in the neck.

Newer vehicles have the headrest position too far forward for many drivers, which actually pushes the driver's head forward and causes neck/back pain, headaches and driver distraction. Adjustment controls are the most frequently cited problem for headrest issues.

As of 2009, National Highway Traffic Safety Administration safety standards designed to reduce whiplash injuries in rear-end collisions went into effect. These standards established a higher minimum height requirement for front seats and a requirement limiting the distance between the back of an occupant's head and the headrest. The headrest is to be a distance of 2.2 inches or less from the back of the head.

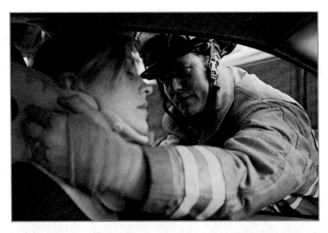

So if you have a vehicle with a model year prior to 2009, we suggest you make sure your headrest is adjusted to the proper height. For those who own cars purchased after 2009 we suggest you continue adjusting to a point of comfort. The positive to come out of all of this is that there is an attention to detail to protect the occupant's neck without causing discomfort in the process.

Oftentimes an ounce of prevention is worth a pound of cure. Benjamin Franklin said that it is better to keep a bad thing from happening then to fix the bad thing once it has happened. That is why it is so important to stay healthy now and prevent injury rather than deal with a lengthy treatment program and an undefined outcome.

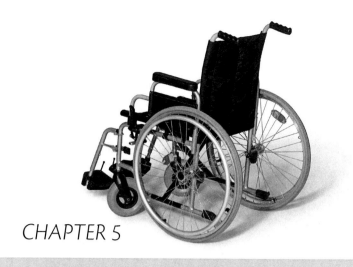

CHAPTER 5

FIRST AID FOR NECK AND BACK PAIN

ortunately, most cases of neck and back pain get better by taking anti-inflammatories like aspirin or ibuprofen and getting off your feet. Voltaire once wrote "The only purpose of the physician is to amuse the patient while nature cures the disease." Along this vein of thinking, home remedies are often successful for the most common cause of neck and back pain — simple muscle strain.

Home Remedy #1: Stop What You Are Doing

Pain is a symptom of an injury, so kick back and relax. A few pillows under your knees and a thin foam pillow for the neck are in order. You can lay on your side with a pillow between your knees. Only 24 hours rest is appropriate.

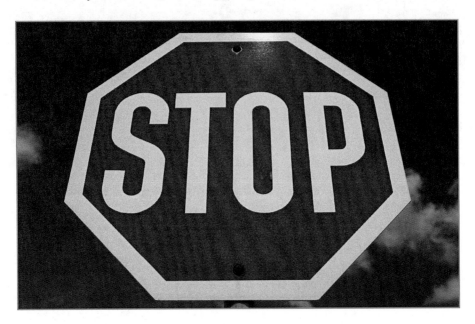

Home Remedy #2: Over-the-Counter Nonsteroidal Anti-Inflammatories (NSAIDs)

Aspirin, ibuprofen and naproxen are nonsteroidal anti-inflammatories that help decrease swelling in the muscles. Start the medicine right after injury, take the smallest effective dose and remember to take it with food.

Home Remedy #3: Ice Then Heat

Use ice for the first 24 hours. Place the ice in a plastic bag and wrap a pillow case or towel around it. Apply to the injured area for 20 minute periods at a time. After 24 hours, use heat; either warm Turkish towels or a heating pad. Be careful not to lay directly on the heat and burn yourself.

Home Remedy #4: Topical Analgesics

Topical analgesic products (e.g. creams, transdermal patches etc.) are of benefit for superficial pain relief. This often plays a distractive role.

Home Remedy #5: Massage

Oftentimes a good massage will stretch out tight muscles and ligaments.

Home Remedy #6: Exercise

Start out with a walking program. Just getting the blood flowing will often stimulate the body's own painkillers, beta-endorphins. Flexion or extension-based exercise programs may be helpful after determining which of the two gives the best pain relief.

Home Remedy #7: Modify

Employ proper body mechanics, modify how you position your body in space, and avoid sitting for prolonged periods of time, driving long distances, and lifting anything heavy.

Home Remedy #8: Think Calming Thoughts

Stress and anxiety increase pain, so learning to de-stress can actually accelerate healing.

Home Remedy #9: Sex and Recreational Exercise

It is important that sex and recreational needs continue during recovery, but creative modification is important to avoid re-injury.

Danger Signs

Usually, neck or back pain gets better in one to two days with rest and NSAIDs. If the pain gets worse, there is loss of bowel or bladder control, or loss of strength in your arms or legs, see a spine specialist or go to the emergency room ASAP.

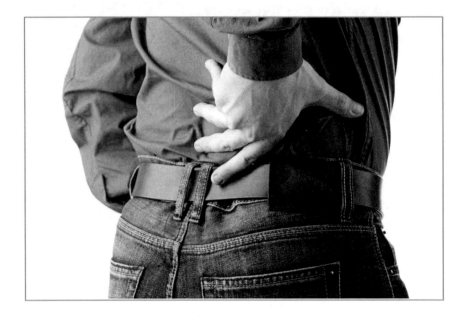

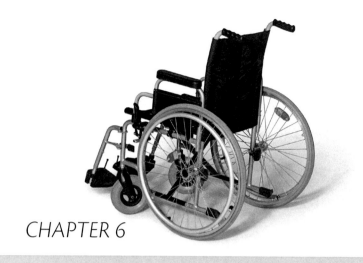

CHAPTER 6

NONOPERATIVE TREATMENT

Whenever you sustain an injury or begin to develop signs or symptoms of dysfunction, you should have an assessment. Most neck and back symptoms respond to general first aid. But if symptoms do not respond in five to seven days, you should see a doctor for an assessment. There are, of course, situations where an urgent evaluation should be performed. Motor vehicle accidents, falls from a great height, and spontaneous onset of neurologic symptoms such as numbness, tingling, pain or paralysis all warrant immediate evaluations, but elective assessments should also be obtained for those with low-grade symptoms, symptoms of long-term duration and those not involving any neurologic deficits.

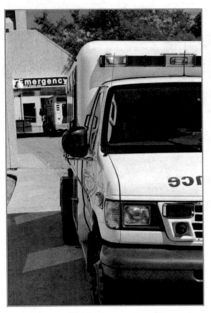

After an assessment is performed, nonoperative or conservative treatment may come in the form of medications (topical, oral or injectable), therapies, orthoses or modalities. The decision regarding which type of treatment to pursue is dependent on the experience and training of the provider and the signs/symptoms of the patient. It should be remembered that all treatments have a potential for side effects and/or complications, so it is often prudent to begin with the safest and progress to the more invasive treatments or those with more known side effects only if needed.

Prescription Pain Medications

Prescription medications come in the form of narcotics, muscle relaxers, corticosteroids, depressants, and anti-seizure medications that help modulate the sensation of pain.

Narcotic or opioid pain relievers should only be used for severe pain and for short periods of time. The use of narcotics for more than three to four weeks is not recommended. Narcotics block the feeling of pain and can result in abuse, dependency or addiction. Some prescription narcotics include:

- Codeine
- Fentanyl — available as a patch
- Hydrocodone
- Hydromorphone

- Morphine
- Oxycodone
- Tramadol

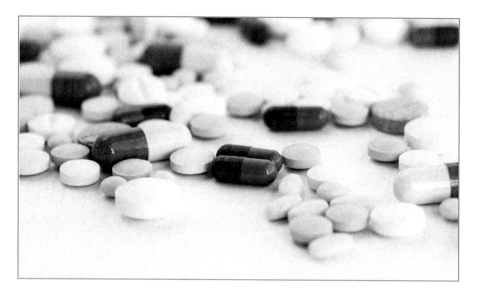

Muscle relaxers relax contracted muscles but can be extremely sedating. Carisoprodol may be more addictive than others. Some muscle relaxers include:

- Cyclobenzaprine
- Diazepam
- Methocarbamol
- Baclophen
- Clonazepam
- Dantrolene
- Tizanidine

In some patients who do not respond to oral medications, local injections of onabotulinumtoxinA or abotulinumtoxin, deep brain stimulation, or the implantation of a baclofen pump may be required.

Antidepressants work by changing certain levels of chemicals in your brain and thus changing the way your brain notices pain. Generally, antidepressants are used for chronic pain situations and include:

- Amitriptyline
- Desipramine
- Duloxetine
- Imipramine
- Nortriptyline

Anti-seizure and anticonvulsant medications are also effective for the treatment of pain. The following medications change the electric signals in your brain and work best for pain that is caused by nerve damage:

- Carbamazepine
- Gabapentin
- Lamotrigine
- Pregabalin
- Valproic acid

All of these drugs have their own side effects. Common side effects include weight gain or weight loss, loss of appetite, upset stomach, rashes, drowsiness or feelings of confusion and headaches. Do not take these drugs unless you are under a doctor's care. Do not stop these drugs suddenly or change dosage without discussing it with your physician.

Injectable pain medications should only be used as a last resort as there are greater chances for dependency and addiction. Overdose is a major concern.

Topical Pain Medications

- Local anesthetics (lidocaine patches)
- Pain medications (anti-inflammatory drugs, narcotic pain relievers and topical pain relievers)
- Counterirritants (contain menthol, eucalyptus, or oil of wintergreen)

Do not use a topical pain reliever if the skin is not normal (such as an open wound or rash). Avoid applying too much as overdose is possible.

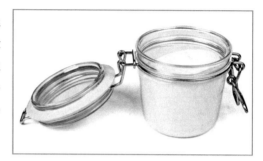

Medications For Inflammation

Medications used to manage inflammation of the musculoskeletal system either caused by arthritis or other disorders are usually categorized into either steroidal or nonsteroidal anti-inflammatory medications. The use of these medications can cause serious side effects including stomach ulcers and bleeding. Also these medications may be harmful when used with blood thinning medicines and alcohol.

Nonsteroidal anti-inflammatory drugs (NSAIDs) are used to manage pain and inflammation. Commonly used NSAIDs include aspirin, ibuprofen, naproxen, diclofenac and celecoxib. When a body part is inflamed, it secretes prostaglandins, which result in inflammation, pain, swelling and fever/warmth. NSAIDs block the specific enzyme used by the body to make prostaglandins, which helps relieve the symptoms.

Common side effects of NSAIDs include:

- Elevated liver enzymes
- Diarrhea
- Headache
- Dizziness
- Hypertension
- Salt and fluid retention
- Ulcers

A stronger type of anti-inflammatory medication is the oral steroid category. Oral steroids come in many forms but are usually ordered as a Medrol Dosepak. The dose pack starts with a high dose and then tapers down to a lower dose over the course of five to six days. When used on a short-term basis there are generally few complications. Side effects include stomach ulcers, weight gain, osteoporosis, avascular necrosis of the hip joints and others. It is advised that diabetics not use oral steroids as they may dramatically increase blood sugars. Patients with an active infection should also avoid steroid use.

Other Types of Medication

Herbal medications are derived from plants that are used medicinally to treat health problems. Many herbs are felt to provide decreased inflammation and help manage pain. Yet caution should be exercised as these herbs not only have the potential to help, but also may have the potential to harm through side effects, allergic reactions and interactions with others substances or medications.

Herbal pain relief medications:

- Capsaicin

- Ginger
- Feverfew
- Turmeric
- Devil's claw

Herbs for pain management:

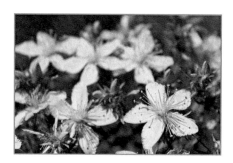

- Ginseng
- Kava kava
- St. John's Wort
- Valerian root

It should be noted that safety and efficacy research is still limited regarding the use of herbal therapies for pain management. The government does not regulate herbal products for quality. The best course of action is to talk to a health professional before testing out one of these herbal remedies. Certainly before any surgery, tell your physician and surgeon what you are taking and be prepared to stop two weeks prior to surgery.

Physical Therapy

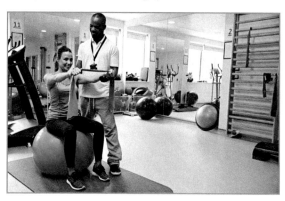

Physical therapy is performed by a trained physical therapist to evaluate your injury or level of impairment, formulate a treatment plan and provide a manual treatment for those with dysfunction. Physical therapy may involve methods such as heat, ice, transcutaneous electrical nerve stimulation (TENS) and/or low-level laser therapy for the treatment of localized symptoms. Additionally, range of motion, strengthening, coordination of muscle use, gait training and balance may be required for those with injury and/or neurologic deficit.

Weight loss is important to decrease the load carried by your joints. Take for example your knees; your knees carry four times your body weight. So if you weigh 180 pounds the normal pressure on your knees is 720 pounds. Say you then lose 20 pounds. Then the pressure on your knees drops down to 640. Ideally you should keep your weight within a healthy range with a BMI (body mass index) of 18.5 to 24.9.

Lastly, protecting your joints can help you control your daily arthritis joint pain. When standing or walking, don't stand too long in one place, keep your feet wide apart to distribute your weight evenly and ditch the high heels. When sitting or resting, change positions frequently. When performing material handling, lift objects with your legs, and avoid excessive squatting or kneeling.

Whether it is a hip joint, a knee joint, a finger joint, or a spine joint, the principles are the same. The only difference with spine joints is that there are more risks inherent, as one must have concerns for protecting the spinal cord and nerve roots; they are not replaceable and result in significant impairment when damaged.

In 1981, Robin McKenzie a physical therapist from New Zealand introduced the McKenzie method for patients with neck and low back pain. His method involves three steps, consisting of evaluation, treatment and prevention. In the evaluation phase a patient undergoes repeated movements and sustained positions. During this period of time a pattern of pain responses called centralization is identified. Based on this evaluation an exercise program is designed based upon the direction of pain initiation — whether pain occurs during flexion (bending), extension or lateral shift (moving side to side). The aim of the therapy is to reduce pain, centralize the symptoms or concentrate them out of the arm or leg into the neck or the small of the low back and then completely recover from the pain. Once this progression of maneuvers is identified, the program consists of educating and encouraging the patient to exercise regularly and perform self care.

When extension is as the directional preference, the patient usually begins in the prone lying position and progresses to a push-up position. When flexion is the directional preference, patients began lying on their back progressing to knees on chest, bending over and then eventually touching their toes.

Generally an extension program is of benefit for a patient with a disc lesion, whereas a flexion program is more beneficial for a patient with spinal stenosis. If you want personal guidance on this exercise program, is consult a physical therapist who has completed the McKenzie therapy training courses.

Pool-based therapy

Back pain can have a number of causes so the first thing to do is to get a careful evaluation and diagnosis by your spine specialist. If physical therapy is recommended it may either be land-based or in the pool.

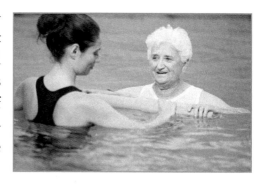

Some reasons a physical therapist might recommend pool-based therapy is if the patient has the following issues:

- Severe deconditioning
- Weight-bearing intolerance or the inability to stand and walk
- Multiple arthritic joints

Pool therapy may include swimming, water walking, unloading exercises with buoyancy vests or water jogging. Swimming is an excellent form of low-impact cardio conditioning. Most weight-bearing exercises, such as running, exert high levels of stress on the spine. Swimming has practically no impact on spinal structures, as the water is able to support the body relieving stresses on all joints. Swimming may also strengthen the neck, back and core muscles.

The most popular strokes are:

- **Backstroke** – Minimizes spinal stress and is ideal for patients with weak abdominal muscles.
- **Freestyle** – May increase neck and back pain, especially during breathing.
- **Breaststroke** – A favored stroke for patients with spine problems.

Swimming may cause neck or back pain if you are in a hyperextended position, such as during a front crawl, butterfly or breaststroke, or if the stroke you are doing requires hyperextension of the neck to breathe.

If you are trying to lose weight by beginning an exercise program, you may consider using a treadmill or elliptical. Both can be particularly useful pieces of equipment for the obese, but not all ellipticals and treadmills are built to hold a lot of weight. A treadmill generally has a weight capacity of 400 pounds, whereas an elliptical trainer usually has a weight capacity of 300 pounds. In general, treadmills hold more weight than ellipticals. All this must be considered when designing a program for the morbidly obese.

The incorporation of therapeutic exercise into a rehabilitation program is extremely important unless your physician directs otherwise. Therapeutic exercise helps to reduce pain and increases function in nearly all musculoskeletal injuries. But not all rehabilitation programs are the same. Occasionally a program is not successful. If that appears to be the way you are heading, here are some suggestions to prevent failure.

Here are some considerations to explain program failure:

- Inaccurate initial assessment
- Lack of secondary assessments
- Poor exercise techniques
- Lack of multidisciplinary approach
- Poor supervision
- Lack of modification of exercise for progression
- Outdated techniques
- Poor engagement

Braces

Braces have been developed to immobilize various areas of the spine. A cervical brace may take the form of a soft collar, halo, Philadelphia collar or cervicothoracic brace such as a Minerva or SOMI brace. The Philadelphia collar is the most common form of cervi-

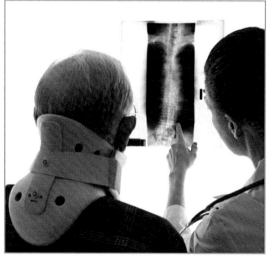

cal orthosis. It is used by EMTs on the street after acute trauma in order to immobilize the cervical spine, and it is used for patients who sustain spinal injuries. The Philadelphia collar is a stiff foam collar composed of two pieces that are attached at the sides with

Velcro straps. The Philadelphia collar is extremely effective at limiting motion in the mid-cervical spine area and is frequently used after cervical spine surgery. It is also used to stabilize minor cervical spinal fractures and to reduce pain associated with a muscular strain. A halo is the most rigid cervical brace and is best for upper cervical lesions. Thoracolumbar, lumbar and lumbosacral braces may be used to immobilize areas of the chest and/or abdominal/pelvic areas.

Braces may be used to treat soft tissue or bony injuries. The length of use is dependent upon the magnitude of the injury, the neurologic deficit and the stability needed you return to mobility.

Alternatively, lumbar supports or binders are divided into lumbar supports and lumbosacral supports. The lumbar support provides support to the lumbar or low back area whereas the lumbosacral support provides support to both the lumbar and sacral or upper buttocks areas. For people who have injury or illness or lack the ability to maintain proper posture on their own for longer periods of time, a binder is a good idea. For people who work in a job that require lifting or other strenuous exercise a back binder can reduce the risk of back injury. Back binders should only be worn during periods of strenuous exercise or activities.

Belly wraps

What's a belly wrap? A belly wrap is a product that claims to aid people to lose abdominal weight faster during a workout. The claim is that the belly wrap heats up the midsection area during a workout, which is supposed to target weight loss in that area. There are claims that people have lost weight and decreased waist size by using these wraps.

The reality is that weight loss is achieved not from losing fat but merely by fluid loss from excessive sweating. After the workout when one rehydrates the weight immediately returns. The danger of these bodysuits or body wraps is that excessive sweat can leave you susceptible to overheating, resulting in dizziness, weakness and mental confusion.

Treatment Modalities

Ice and heat

Patients always ask physicians if they should use heat or ice on an injured or painful area of their body. As a general rule it is often recommended that ice be used for the first 24 hours of pain to decrease pain and swelling, but heat be used thereafter to increase circulatory flow and promote healing.

The facts are that there is some evidence that heat will decrease low back pain, but there is little proof that cold will help. Patients will need to decide which feels more beneficial to them.

How to use ice for low back pain:

- Use ice in a plastic bag covered by a towel, an ice pack, or a bag of frozen vegetables
- Ice area three times a day for approximately 20 minutes
- Ice after vigorous exercise or prolonged activity

How to use heat for low back pain:

- Apply for 15 to 20 minutes at a time
- Moist heat is better than dry heat
- If using a heating pad, be careful to avoid burns
- Pharmacy heat wraps may also be beneficial

Try alternating:

- Use heat for 15 to 20 minutes, then ice for 10 to 15 minutes

TENS

Transcutaneous electrical nerve stimulation (TENS) is a device that uses electric current to stimulate nerves for therapeutic purposes. Electrical stimulation for pain has been known since 63 A.D. in ancient Rome. Benjamin Franklin was also a proponent of this method for pain relief. The modern TENS unit is credited to C. Norman Shealy.

The TENS unit is used as a noninvasive nerve stimulation for both acute and chronic pain. There is some evidence that it is useful for pain, yet there is other evidence which does not support the use of TENS for chronic low back pain. Recent studies have suggested that patients with acute complete spinal cord injury may develop recovery of motor function with the use of transcutaneous electrical stimulation. It appears that the stimulation causes a reawakening of nerve connections.

LLLT

Low-level laser therapy (LLLT), also known as cold laser therapy or photobiomodulation, is the application of light to promote tissue repair, reduce inflammation, induce analgesia or relieve pain. Think of a light going through a prism and all the colors of the rainbow coming out. In the electromagnetic spectrum light is made of various colors. The different colors represent wavelengths of light that are in a spectrum ranging from microwave to infrared to near infrared to visible light to ultraviolet to X-rays. Each laser of light has a different effect.

LLLT takes specific wavelengths of light and projects them through the skin to get specific effects. Think of LLLT like photosynthesis in plants. Just as sunshine is necessary for plants to grow and stay healthy, so can we use light for pain relief.

There were 30 papers on LLLT published in 2012 and there have been over 300 clinical trials and 3000 laboratory studies on LLLT. There are also several ongoing studies at Harvard. The device is FDA approved and is also approved in Europe and Canada.

The four common clinical targets for LLLT are:

1. Site of injury to promote healing, remodeling and reduce inflammation
2. Lymph nodes to reduce swelling and inflammation
3. Induction of analgesia or pain relief
4. Trigger points to reduce tenderness and relax contracted muscles

The number of treatments required is dependent on several variables. The faster an injury is treated, the faster it resolves. But remember that if the treatment is started and not completed, oftentimes the pain returns worse than before, just like stopping antibiotics before an infection is cleared.

LLLT is used by high-level amateur and professional athletes worldwide. With this new technology patients can relieve pain and heal injuries without surgery, injections, pain medications, or stomach ulcers.

Steroid injections and other injection therapy

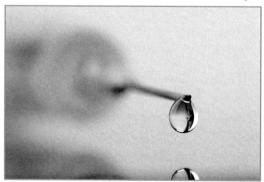

Epidural steroid injections is a technique for relieving pain using a needle, local anesthetic and corticosteroids. The medication is injected into the epidural space surrounding a nerve or the spinal cord. The anesthetic results in short-term pain relief and the corticosteroids give longer-term relief. It is believed the corticosteroids have an anti-inflammatory effect on the neural structures.

Epidural steroid injections are controversial. Most studies conclude the pain relief from such injections are primarily a result of the anesthetic and do not reduce the need for surgical care.

Epidural steroid injections are performed with fluoroscopy and a radio-opaque contrast agent so that medication may be accurately placed. After the treatment the patient may get up and walk immediately and gradually resume normal activities.

Candidates for epidural steroid injections include patients with the following conditions:

- Spinal stenosis
- Spondylolisthesis
- Spondylolysis
- Herniated disc
- Degenerative disc
- Sciatica

Risk from an epidural steroid injection include spinal headache, bleeding, infection, allergic reaction, nerve damage /paralysis. The side effects from include weight gain, water retention, flushing, mood swings, insomnia and elevated blood sugar in diabetics.

Recent studies demonstrate that epidural steroid injections may offer temporary relief of sciatica, but based on systematic reviews these injections do not reduce the rate of subsequent required surgery. Despite the limited benefit of epidural steroid, Medicare claims showed a 271 percent increase over the recent past seven years. For patients with back pain without sciatica there is no evidence of benefit from these injections. Recent studies have shown that in patients with lumbar spinal stenosis, epidural steroid injections are less effective than local analgesic injections.

The injection of steroids into a local area is a method used by physicians to treat inflammation. Steroid injections are often injected directly into a joint to treat conditions such as gout, rheumatoid arthritis or other inflammatory diseases. Steroids may also be injected into other joints such as the shoulder, elbow, hip, knee, hand or wrist, as well as around tendons.

More recently Synvisc-One (hylan G-F 20) (Sanofi, Bridgewater, New Jersey) has been introduced for the treatment of pain associated with osteoarthritis of the knee. For those patients who have not had success with conservative nonpharmacologic therapy and analgesics such as Tylenol, injection therapy may be necessary. Synvisc-One was designed to cushion and lubricate the knees. Synvisc-One is a naturally occurring substance called hyaluronic acid and is found in rooster combs. Synvisc-One is chemically modified to increase its molecular weight and requires a series of three doses. Another similar injection therapy is Hyalgan (hyaluronic acid) (Fidia Pharma USA Inc, Parsippany, New Jersey) which is not chemically modified and requires five doses.

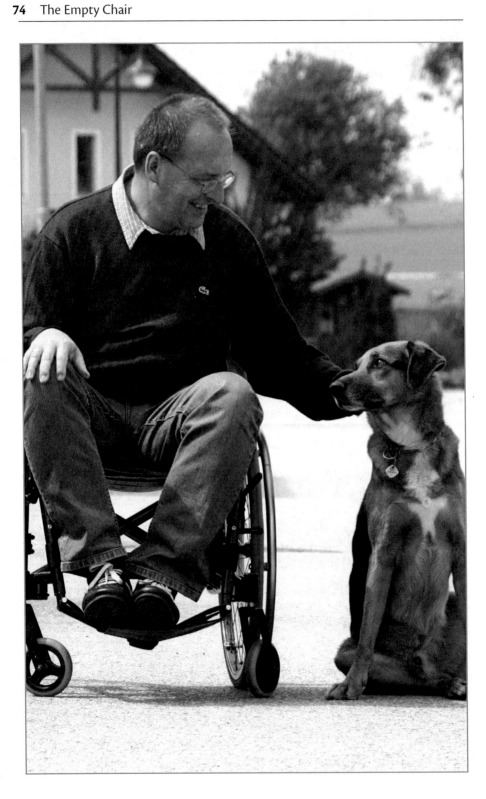

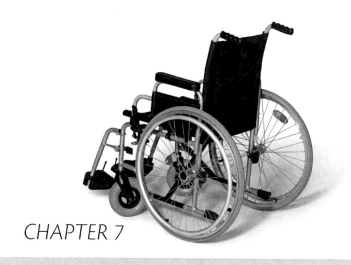

CHAPTER 7

WHEELCHAIR EXERCISES AND LIMITED MOBILITY FITNESS

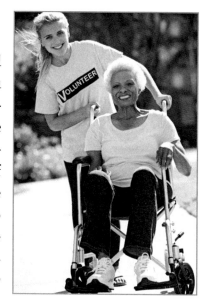

Just because you have limited mobility does not mean you are unable to exercise. Exercise is important to build muscle mass, relieve stress, ease depression and anxiety, restore a sense of worth or self-esteem, and improve your outlook on life. Those who have an impairment due to severe weight problems, osteoarthritis, paralysis, stroke, diabetes or any other form of chronic illness can benefit from some form of exercise. Exercise can help you overcome some physical limitations, aid your caretakers and restore a more positive outlook on life. Just because you are not able to walk and cannot partake in all the various forms of sports or exercise that are available to those who are ambulatory does not mean you cannot find an enjoyable way to exercise. When people exercise they release a beta-endorphin, which is able to inhibit pain and generate a sense of well-being. Why do you think the marathoner is able to run in spite of having sores and blisters all over his or her feet? The answer is beta-endorphins. Those who have sustained an injury, are inactive due to chronic disease, frail due to aging or have a fear of injury need to develop techniques to overcome their immobility issues and learn to benefit physically, mentally and emotionally from exercise.

THE FOUR ESSENTIALS OF EXERCISE

It is important to remember the four essentials of exercise:

1. Cardiovascular
2. Core strengthening
3. Strength training
4. Flexibility

Whether you are wheelchair dependent or not, it is important to remember that each type of exercise is important to overcome obstacles or deficiencies. Cardiovascular exercise is important to raise your heart rate and your health in general. Any exercise that has the potential to increase your heart rate is considered cardio. Walking, dancing, cycling, swimming, water aerobics and aqua jogging are all types of cardio.

Core strengthening is important in order to have better sitting posture in the wheelchair. You must be creative when developing exercises based on the neurology and muscle availability.

Strength training involves the use of weights or elastic bands that generate a resistance and allow you to build muscle and bone mass, prevent falls and improve balance. The increased inactivity associated with wheelchair dependence results in muscle atrophy. Without strength training, a wheelchair dependent will require additional aid for the activities of daily living.

Flexibility exercises are important to reduce pain and stiffness, prevent falls and/or injury and improve range of motion. Yoga and stretching exercises can aid in preventing or delaying additional muscle atrophy.

Now, how do you get started when you have limited mobility? First you have to develop a routine. Every day you have to say to yourself, "I'm going to make myself better today." Start slow and gradually increase your activity level. Incorporate your exercise routine into your daily life. Stay committed to your goal and make it a habit. Your goal is to try to have a better life with improved mood, less stress and a longer life then you would have without exercising. Be sure to understand that you will have good days and bad days. Do not be afraid to skip a day if you have an injury, or if you just do not feel like exercising that day. But remember, momentum is your friend. Once you get started it is important that you stay safe while exercising. Wear comfortable clothing, stay hydrated, warm up, stretch, cool down, avoid exercise or activity involving an injured body part and stop exercising if you feel pain.

In addition to physical challenges one may experience emotional or mental barriers to exercising. Some people feel self-conscious about working out in a crowded gym when they are overweight, have a disability, have sustained an injury or illness. This is when the "poor, poor, pitiful me syndrome" starts to appear. If this happens it is important to realize it, explain it to family and friends, and ask for support and encouragement. Also, it is important to be entertained and engaged while you exercise, so do things you think will be fun. Think of the three Es — **entertain, engage and exercise**.

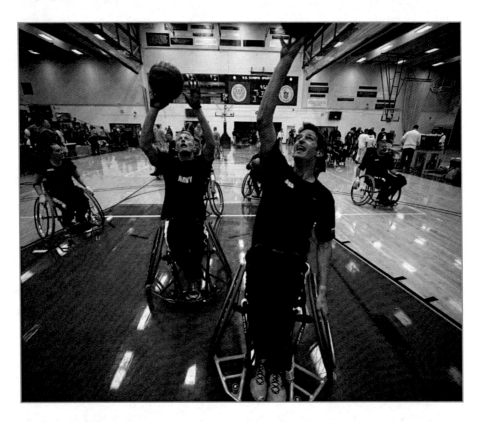

The U.S. Department of Health and Human Services recommends that adults with disabilities should attempt at least 150 minutes moderate intensity cardio a week or 75 minutes a week of vigorous intensity cardio exercise with each workout lasting at least 10 minutes. Two or more sessions a week of moderate or high intensity strength training activities should also be performed.

The bottom line is if you are unable to meet this requirement due to your abilities you should at least avoid complete inactivity.

Some wheelchair dependent people can still walk, jog, swim, and use an elliptical machine or treadmill. If you have limitations consider a recumbent bike or an upper extremity bike for your cardio exercise. Injury or disability may limit weightlifting, but it is still important to try. If you are unable to do your lower extremities then just work with what you have got. Isometric exercise will also help you maintain muscle strength and prevent deterioration. An exercise program involving a chair or wheelchair can be modified.

For those patients suffering from obesity, diabetes and all the comorbidities associated with being overweight, it is important to start an exercise program. Special equipment is available and activity monitors can be extremely useful. It is important to incorporate your activity program into everyday life. The four essentials of exercise still apply.

In addition to regular exercise there are aerobic exercises, yoga and Pilates, which are known as **sitting aerobics**. These exercises will improve posture and reduce spine pain. These exercises also focus on upper body movements and improve overall fitness.

Yoga is an expression of uniqueness. Through yoga, those who are wheelchair dependent may also express their individuality.

The benefits of wheelchair yoga include:

- Restful sleep
- Decreased isolation
- Feelings of well-being
- Decreased tension stress and anxiety
- Improved focus

- Increased lung capacity
- Greater strength
- Improved flexibility

The following yoga poses may be performed in a wheelchair:

- Cat pose
- Cow pose
- Side stretch
- Hip stretch
- Leg stretch
- Twist
- Eagle pose
- Forward bend

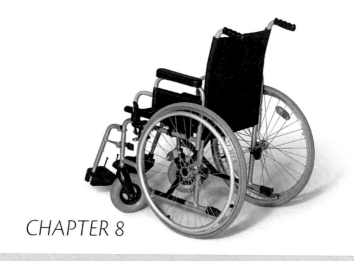

CHAPTER 8

OPERATIVE TREATMENT

M aking a decision can be difficult. Fear of making the wrong decision can be punishing. Failure to make the correct decision may be due to poor decision-making methodology. Gut instincts can only take you so far in life.

In order to learn how to make the correct decision regarding surgery, you need to learn how to synthesize an overwhelming amount of incoming information and to make the best decision in a time-

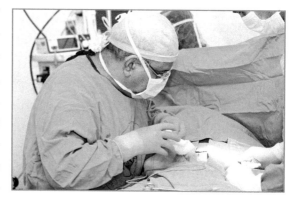

ly fashion. The best way to take a volume of information, synthesize it and make a decision is to learn how to deal with the hierarchy of knowledge.

Hierarchy of knowledge:

1. Gut instincts
2. Data
3. Information
4. Knowledge

MAKING A DECISION WITHOUT REGRET

When it comes time to make a big life decision, such as having surgery, consider the following seven steps of making a decision without regret:

1. Have a life vision
2. Evaluate the pros and cons
3. Discuss with a friend
4. Invoke a higher power
5. Flip a coin, but decide what you would choose before the flip
6. Ask questions
7. Don't regret

Most people do not want to have surgery. It is natural for people to wish and hope that their condition is self-limiting and will resolve itself relatively quickly. There are occasions when procrastination can result in a worsening of the condition and make correction more difficult. If someone finds themselves in this situation it is important to be educated about the problem, find a physician you feel comfortable with and consider a second opinion. Prompt decisions can prevent irreversible damage.

Spinal surgery may have one of three objectives — decompression, stabilization and/or ablation. Decompressive spinal surgery is designed to take the pressure off a neural structure, while stabilization of the spine is performed to restore stability lost either from an injury or a decompression surgery. Ablation is performed to remove, negate or destroy a structure such as a disc, nerve or tumor. Traditionally these surgeries have been performed by large open incisions but more recently, minimally invasive spinal surgery has been introduced.

Minimally invasive spine surgery is the new in thing in spinal surgery. Performing minimally invasive spine surgery is like building a ship in a bottle. The term minimally invasive describes surgical procedures that are performed through small incisions or openings to gain access to a specific part of the body. The purpose of minimally invasive surgery is to reduce damage to surrounding tissues, speed up healing and recover with less pain.

Advantages:

- Quicker return to activities
- Smaller incision
- Less damage to surrounding muscle
- Potentials for less blood loss, shorter hospital stay, quicker healing and potentially less pain

Disadvantages:

- Steep learning curve
- Potential for prolonged operative times
- Increased radiation exposure
- Not appropriate for every case
- Difficult to apply bone for fusion cases
- Difficult to repair a spinal fluid leak

Minimally invasive techniques for spine surgery have been used since the 1990s predominantly for decompressions and limited fusions. Newer techniques are currently being developed to push the envelope and perform internal fixation, but remember that it is still spine surgery.

Outpatient, or ambulatory, surgery is very common in orthopedic surgery. Historically it has occurred in hand, foot and sports medicine surgeries. Now with the introduction of newer medications, surgical techniques and accelerated recovery programs, this innovation has allowed a movement to outpatient surgery for joint replacement and spinal surgery. Spinal surgical procedures that are conducive to outpatient procedures are smaller cases such as laminectomies, disectomies, foraminotomies, one level anterior cervical fusions, one level transforaminal lumbar interbody fusions, and one level decompression/stabilization procedures.

In order to be a candidate you must be:

- Physiologically younger
- Healthy
- More active
- Motivated
- Able to play hurt

There is currently a greater emphasis on performing less invasive surgeries while trying to mobilize the patient as rapidly as possible. Patient selection is important. Those patients who require more extensive procedures, have medical comorbidities, or require careful postoperative monitoring, will continue to need traditional inpatient hospital settings.

In order to decrease cost, expense, lost time from work, and have a safe procedure, it is important to educate yourself about ambulatory surgery and plan carefully.

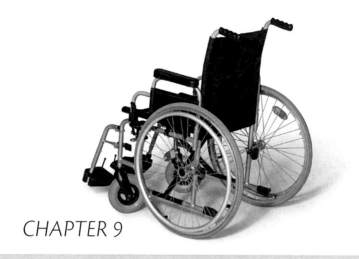

PREVENTION

P redicting how life expectancy is affected by a medical condition is nearly impossible. Still there are factors that may affect a person's life expectancy.

The following are a list of impairments and key disabilities which are factors which may help to predict a shorter life expectancy.

- severity of illness
- mobility restrictions
- feeding difficulties
- seizures
- cognitive functioning
- visual acuity

- respiratory function
- cardiac status

When one evaluates a senior's walking speed, along with age and gender, one is now able to predict life expectancy. **Gait or walking is a powerful indicator of vitality.** The ability to walk takes into consideration circulatory, respiratory, skeletal, muscular and nervous systems. So if one of these systems is impaired then it will eventually affect life expectancy. A spinal condition which impairs one's ability to walk will thus have a negative effect on life expectancy.

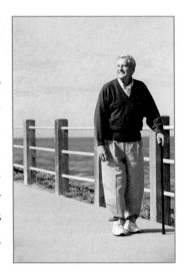

Nutrition

Most people are aware that good nutrition and a balanced diet are important for overall health. Having a healthy life includes preventing problems and healing injuries. The skeleton, its surrounding muscles and other structures need good nutrition, including vitamins, to be strong enough to support the body and perform other functions.

The various roles of vitamins or nutrients:

- **Vitamin A –** For the immune system, tissue repair and bone formation.
- **Vitamin B12 –** For bone marrow

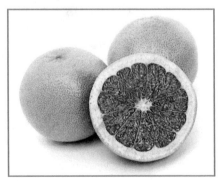

- **Vitamin C** – For collagen development, which allows tissue to heal
- **Vitamin D** – Develops strong and healthy bones
- **Vitamin K** – Helps bones stay strong and healthy
- **Iron** – Needed for hemoglobin and myoglobin transport
- **Magnesium** – Important for muscle function and bone density
- **Calcium** – Essential for bone health

Exercise is important to build muscle mass. But how can you gain more muscle mass with less time for training? The secret is in nutrition.

Here is a list of the top 10 foods to build muscle mass.

1. Lean beef
2. Skinless chicken
3. Cottage cheese
4. Fish
5. Whey protein
6. Eggs
7. Oatmeal
8. Fruits and vegetables
9. Whole grains
10. Healthy fats including nuts, flaxseed oil, avocados and seeds

If you are trying to lose weight there are foods that you must avoid:

- Frozen meals
- High-fiber bars
- Any all carbs snack

- Juices
- Low-fat foods
- Alcohol
- Artificially sweetened drinks
- Supersized snacks or cereal
- Fast foods
- Fried foods
- Cakes and cookies
- Candy
- Ice cream sugar, honey and jams
- Breads and pastas

Nicotine

Remember that first puff of a cigarette? The wave of nausea, the dizziness, the cough, the lightheadedness? This is the smoker's high. Why do some put the 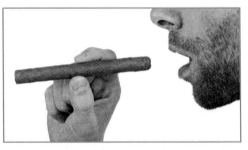 cigarettes down and never pick them up again while others become physically and psychologically addicted?

In spite of it being a known fact that cigarettes cause cancer, heart disease, emphysema, and other diseases, 20 percent of the American population continues to smoke. Globally four million people die each year from diseases directly related to tobacco.

In cultures that enjoy a longer life expectancy, the disease, as a result of the accumulation of bodily insult and injury, becomes more apparent. Smokers are 2.7 times more likely to have back pain. Smokers develop low back pain as they get older, with women being more prone than men. Smoking is also blamed for the decay of spinal discs, osteoporosis and failure of spinal fusion surgery.

Smoking is responsible for decreased nutrition to the spine due to the carbon monoxide in cigarette smoke. The carbon monoxide sticks to hemoglobin, which is the oxygen carrying part of the blood, and subsequently decreases oxygen supply to all body tissues. Regardless of whether you smoke it, chew it, sniff it or absorb it in a patch, the active substance in tobacco is nicotine. Nicotine, which is the prime chemical in tobacco, increases blood pressure by constricting blood vessels. Nicotine also causes collagen to stop being formed in the center of discs, tendons, ligaments and cartilage. Thus the majority of nonsmokers are able to heal disc lesions. In other relatively avascular structures such as tendons, ligaments and cartilage, these smokers are unable to heal disc tears and other relatively avascular structures. Smokers also have a higher rate of unsuccessful fusions.

Cutting down on smoking decreases the chance of developing back pain and the failure of injury healing. After 48 hours of non-smoking, the nerve endings of your back will start to grow back as a result of the increased blood flow. The cornea of the eye and the intervertebral disc are the only two structures in adult life that do not have a direct blood supply. When smoking cessation occurs, dilatation of the blood vessels and increased blood flow allows for diffusion of nutrients, and results in an increase in oxygen from the bones to the spine to the discs. A disc that is unable to get its nutrition will develop cracks or tears, which will lead to ruptures or herniations.

Your best bet to enjoy good health is to stay active, exercise, and to not smoke or use any other nicotine product.

Safety

Motorcycle helmets save lives. The decrease of closed head injuries from helmet use is noteworthy. Seatbelts have also saved the lives of many of those involved in major motor vehicle accidents. The designs for seatbelts have changed over the years, yet their purpose has not changed. Seatbelts are intended to keep drivers and occupants in position to prevent physical collision with the interior of the motor vehicle.

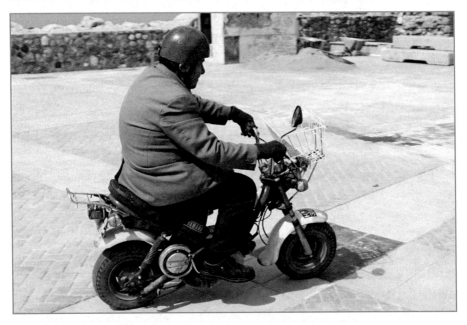

When a collision occurs, the force of impact against another object may stop the vehicle, but the body remains moving at the previous speed. This results in the continued movement of driver and passengers. A dangerous situation can occur if occupants come into contact with the steering wheel, dashboard, windshield, seat or roof of the vehicle. The seatbelt is intended to hold occupants in place and minimize the potential for injury.

Although seatbelts save lives, they may also cause certain injuries. Even when properly fastened and functioning properly, they can result in acute injuries to the neck, shoulders, chest, abdomen and back. Lap belts have been notorious for causing intra-abdominal injury and chance-type spinal fractures.

Preventing Bad Surgery Outcomes

To add insult to injury means to make a bad situation even worse. This statement is the epitome of failed surgery, where someone has a painful condition, has a surgical procedure and feels even worse after.

Failed back surgery syndrome occurs when a surgery to correct pain completely fails to alleviate the pain and in some cases makes the pain even worse. There are many reasons why a surgery could fail to provide results, both related to the patient and the surgeon.

How is it that a patient could cause a surgery to fail? A great example of this would be a patient who has undergone a spinal fusion to correct spinal instability in the lower back. The surgeon has advised the patient that smoking cigarettes could severely reduce the healing chances and affect the fusion process. The patient ignores the doctor and continues to smoke and, as a result, the fusion does not heal. This is a prime example of the patient being at fault.

In what ways could a surgeon be at fault? There are times that there is fault before the surgery is even performed. If there is an inaccurate diagnosis, the surgery could be performed in the wrong area, or the surgery type itself could be wrong. It is important to seek a second opinion from a specialist before proceeding with surgery of any kind. If two heads can agree on what and where the problem is, it is likely that there will be an accurate diagnosis.

One of the most common reasons for failed back surgery syndrome is that the surgeon is just not experienced enough in the technique being performed and as a result, does not perform it properly. This is why it is important to ask your surgeon the right questions before moving forward with the surgery. Be sure to ask how long your surgeon has been performing these surgeries, specifically the procedure you will be undergoing, and how many times a year he or she performs them. If you are not satisfied with any of these answers, find another surgeon. Most surgeries are meant to be a permanent fix for a specific problem and correcting failed surgery is difficult.

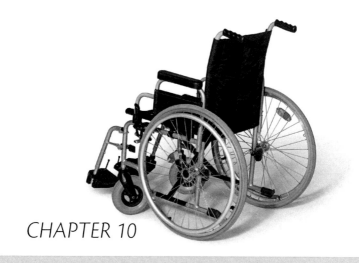

CHAPTER 10

ACCELERATED RECOVERY PROGRAMS

Accelerated recovery programs have been developed for both nonoperative and post-operative patients. When one thinks of speed, one often times thinks of the German autobahn. Just as the German autobahn is fast moving, so is life. The necessity of surgery already puts a damper on your life, so it makes sense that you'd like to spend the least amount of time away from activities during recovery, with the least inconvenience and cost. A Danish surgeon, professor Henrique Kehlet, developed a program in the early 90s to speed up recovery from colorectal surgery. We have taken these principles and applied them to musculoskeletal disorders requiring surgery. Total joint replacement, spine surgery, trauma surgery and surgery of sports injuries need the most assistance for accelerated recovery.

I have developed an accelerated nonoperative and postoperative recovery program for patients undergoing care. Spine surgery is performed to reduce pain, improve function and correct deformity. This program allows you and your surgeon to develop a partnership for your recovery, decreases your injury time, reduces time spent in the hospital, saves you money, increases your comfort, maximizes your recovery, decreases dehydration and starvation, lowers body reaction to stress, and avoids complications. This extensive program involves meticulous preparation and execution in order to obtain early functional recovery and discharge from the hospital. This program can also be used in conjunction with surgical procedures that are specifically designed for accelerated recovery. Everything is carefully planned down to the postoperative dressings, which are flexible, resistant to bacteria, waterproof to allow showering, and made of clear plastic so that the area surrounding the surgical site can be observed. These little details are what make the program successful.

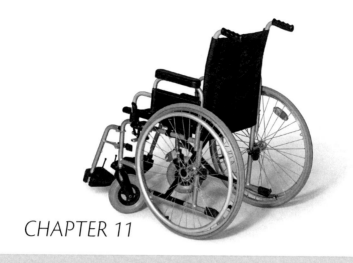

CHAPTER 11

EARLY INTERVENTION

A broken leg is a painful condition. When a leg is broken it is often obvious. So the question is would you continue to run on the broken leg? Or would you take pain medications to mask the pain and then run on it? Or would you just continue with your crutches or wheelchair?

When you sustain an injury your brain tells the injured part of the body that there is pain, to stop and protect that area of the body to allow it to recover. Once the injury has healed the brain has a tendency to hold on to that signal and keep your body in a similar environment to the one you were injured in. Thus the brain feels your body still hurts in spite of it not actually hurting anymore. This is often described as phantom pain. In order to correct the situation you must perform controlled, thoughtful movements so as to break the circuit of phantom pain. In order to prevent re-injury you must perform slow, steady and increasing amounts of exercise. Overdoing it will result in a setback. For the athlete trying to get better faster, a less is more approach is often prudent. Carefully constructing a plan for recovery will avoid setbacks. By consulting your physician or physical therapist or exercise physiologist/trainer you may progress safely through the recovery program.

How to apply the principle:

1. Plan on doing a bit of everything that you had planned for the day
2. Test your movements before excessively loading them
3. Preparation, body and brain warm-up are important

Whenever there is an injury to the central nervous system, whether brain or spinal cord, there is a primary and secondary injury. The primary injury may be evaluated by physical examination and MRI. The MRI gives three patterns of injury that have prognostic value. The first pattern is one of swelling and has the potential for significant recovery. The second pattern is one of hemorrhaging in the brain or spinal cord and has a poor prognosis. The third pattern is a mixed pattern with a combination of swelling and hemorrhaging and has an intermediate recovery potential. Much of the primary damage may be irreversible. Yet this primary injury initiates a cascade of biochemical events that may be reversible. This cascade of biochemical events is known as the secondary injury. If there is mechanical compression on the central nervous system that may benefit from surgical care, then it should be taken care of promptly to maximize recovery. The secondary injury is more amenable to treatment with medical care.

Radiculopathy is the result of a compressed nerve causing pain that radiates into the arm or leg. The compression of the nerve may be either an acute episode, from a whiplash injury, disc herniation or additional traumatic episode such as a fracture. Alternatively radiculopathy can develop over time from a compression of the nerve that is slow and progressive, resulting from thickening of ligaments or arthritis/bone spurs.

The nerve that is affected by radiculopathy comes off of the spinal cord and is called a peripheral nerve. Peripheral nerves have the ability to recover depending upon two factors. One factor is how badly the nerve is compressed and the second factor is the length of time of the compression. Now consider the hit to be very hard or if that nerve is compressed for a long period of time, then the nerve is slow to recover and may not recover completely.

A nerve recovery pattern is not like a light switch where you go from on to off or damaged nerve to normal nerve. There is a period of recovery time. A nerve recovers at the rate of 1 mm per day. Thus one can see that repetitively damaging a nerve results in delayed recovery or inability to recover.

If a nerve is decompressed, the recovery is dependent upon those factors. Usually pain is the first thing that recovers, then weakness, and the last things to recover are numbness/tingling, dysesthesias and exercise intolerance. The recovery of the nerve is variable and depends upon the two injury factors of how badly and how long the nerve has been compressed. If a nerve is not completely and irreversibly damaged there is hope for improvement with decompression.

You should not be sedentary while you are in recovery. You need to get the blood flowing. Getting more blood to the injured area gives it a chance to get healthier.

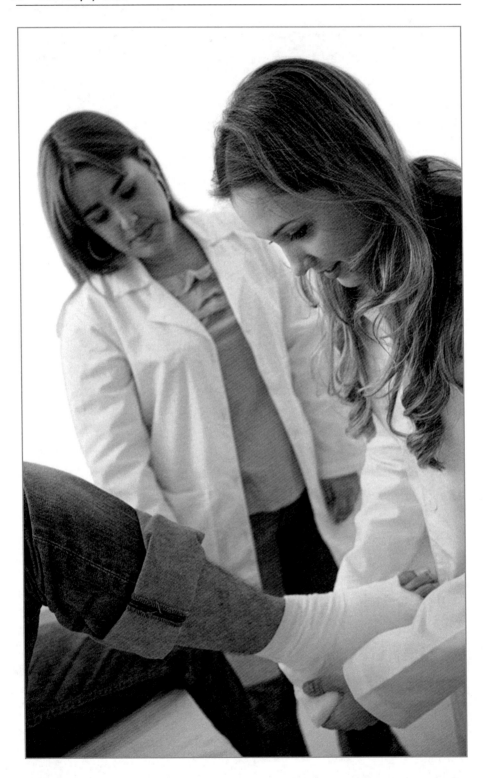

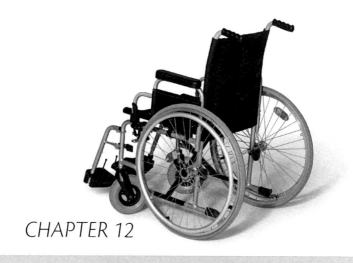

CHAPTER 12

THE TREATERS

C hoosing the right doctor is a big deal. A specialist is a physician who focuses on treating a specific condition exclusively. Why is that so important? Just like any professional athlete, practice makes perfect. And track record is also important as practice usually results in a better outcome.

The word 'doctor' is derived from Latin "docere" which means teacher. For generations, physicians' education has been peer led. The transfer of knowledge is the fabric of the Hippocratic oath. Today that tradition still continues but the method of transfer has changed.

Just as physicians are responsible for educating future physicians, it is also their duty to educate the patient and their family.

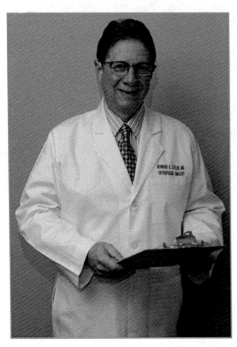

This requires communication. In the era of the electronic medical record, smartphones, computers and other digital devices, physicians have begun directing their focus toward these electronic devices. Medicine is being directed toward a corporate, retail provider model yet the access to medical data is more available than ever before.

In my opinion, in order to improve quality of care, the health care providers need to be unchained from the bureaucracies that strangle them and released to be the teachers they were trained to be. Doctors love educating patients and families about their disease, illness, injury and helping them navigate through the healing process.

A doctor should subscribe to the total transparency manifesto. Patients come to the provider in a time of need. They are scared, vulnerable and in pain. A patient needs to trust that their doctor has their best interest at heart. The patient also needs to know who their doctor is. This relationship is a partnership. Joining in this partnership allows for the creation of a health care system that upholds professionalism, respects human dignity and prioritizes patient values. If you feel uncomfortable with your doctor, get a second opinion and consider a change.

Shared decision-making is a collaborative process that allows patients and their family/advocate to make health care decisions together. By taking into account the best scientific evidence available as well as the patient's values and preferences, the team is usually able to make a good decision.

The first step is to make sure that the provider has the knowledge and communication skills to fully inform the patient of all care options as well as the potential risks and benefits. The second step is to provide the patient with the support of the best individualized care decision. Oftentimes patients make decisions about medical treatments without completely understanding their options or being informed of all their options. The family member or advocate's responsibility is to synthesize the information and aid in the application of the treatment selected.

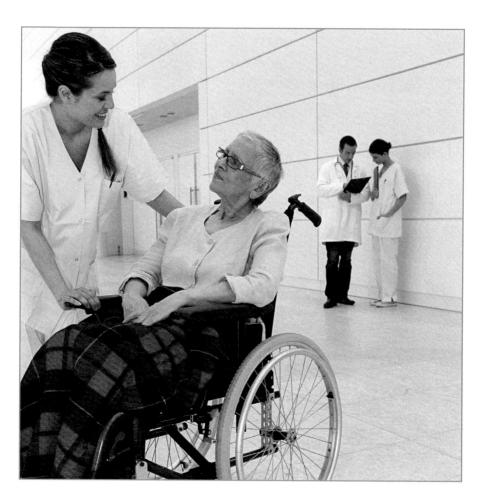

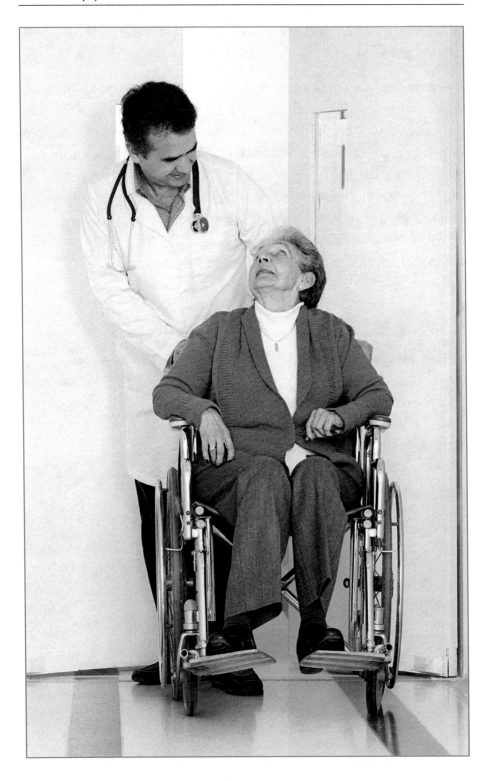

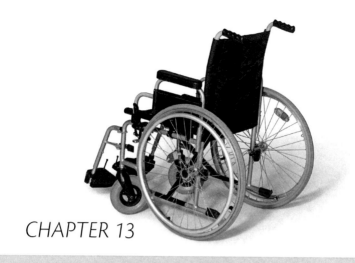

CHAPTER 13

THE DEVICES

D eciding to use a wheelchair is an emotional decision. Most people are reluctant to even think about it. But if your lack of mobility is preventing you from doing things that you want to do and enjoy, then you should consider using a wheelchair. A wheelchair is simply a mobility aid. If you are able to walk at all, walk as much as you are able to safely for exercise. If you have been wheelchair dependent for some time, then be sure to find the most efficient means for mobility.

The wheelchair is simply a chair fitted with wheels. A wheelchair may be either manual or propulsion-based. A manual wheelchair requires the seated occupant to turn the rear wheels by hand, while a propulsion wheelchair is powered by a motor. A wheelchair becomes a necessity for some people who find walking difficult or impossible due to injury, illness, dysfunction or disability.

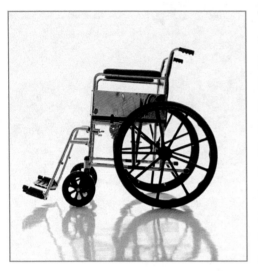

The earliest pictures of wheeled furniture originate in China and Greece around the fifth century BCE. These first portraits depict the disabled being transported in these wheeled devices. But the first true wheelchair used to carry people originates in China around 525 CE. Around 1760, the Bath Chair or invalid carriage began to appear. The Bath Chair was invented by James Heath around 1750 to transport the sick to the waters at the Pump Room or the bath in the Baths. In 1783, James Dawson of Bath, England designed a chair with two large wheels in the back and one small one in the front. Dawson's chair became known as the Bath Chair. The first model wheelchair with rear push wheels and small front casters was patented in 1869. Herbert Everest sustained a broken back in a mining accident and his friend Harry Jennings invented the first lightweight, steel, collapsible wheelchair in 1933. Their x-brace design forms the basis for the first mass manufactured wheelchair.

There are currently many varieties of wheelchairs today. The basic manual wheelchair has a seat, foot rests and four wheels. The two large wheels in the back are used for propulsion as they have hand rims incorporated into the design, while the front caster wheels are smaller for easier navigation. Daily manual wheelchairs are either rigid or folding. The rigid wheelchair was designed for active users who need a more energy-efficient chair to prevent fatigue. The folding wheelchair or transport chair has smaller wheels and was designed to be pushed by a caregiver outside the home. The folding wheelchair is often used in medical settings.

The first motorized wheelchair was manufactured in 1916 in London. Currently electric powered wheelchairs have an electric motor and a joystick that acts as a navigational control. For those who cannot use a manual joystick, sip and puff, chin-operated and head-operated controls are available based on need. These electric power wheelchairs are much more elaborate insofar as their wheeled platform and molded seating system.

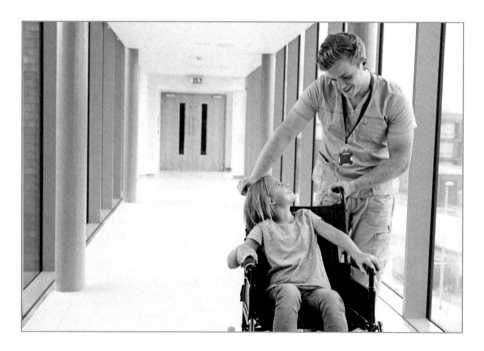

Current wheelchairs come with many options depending upon need. Some of these wheelchairs include:

- Dynamic tilt wheelchairs
- Standing wheelchair
- Bariatric wheelchair

- Pediatric wheelchair
- Knee scooter
- Power assisted wheelchair
- Sports wheelchair
- Stretcher or transfer wheelchair
- All-terrain wheelchair
- Stair climbing wheelchair
- Hand cycle wheelchair
- Stationary wheelchair trainer
- Carbon black wheelchair
- Smart wheelchair

CASE STUDY: STEPHEN HAWKING

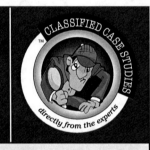

The renowned physicists Stephen Hawking was diagnosed at the age of 21 with amyotrophic lateral sclerosis, also known as Lou Gehrig's disease. He has lived for more than 40 years with the disease, unable to walk, talk, breath, or swallow on his own; he even has difficulty holding his head up. Yet thanks to special modifications made to his wheelchair, he has not only functioned professionally, but thrived in most areas of his life.

In 1963, when Hawking was first diagnosed, he was given a life expectancy of two years by his doctors. While his physical abilities did decline — first he had to use crutches and then lost his ability to write — he found ways to compensate for the abilities he was losing. He eventually accepted the use of a wheelchair in the late 1960s and became a champion for handicap access at facilities and universities in the U.S. and Europe.

Hawking refusal to be limited by his disease and his association with innovative people led him to eventually using a speech synthesizer and a small computer to communicate despite the loss of his voice in 1985.

Hawking has used tools that span from spelling boards, a computer program that allowed users to select words and commands on a screen using a hand clicker, and eventually when his hands grew too weak to use the clicker, a switching device that were attached to his glasses and could detect when Hawking tensed his cheek muscle. This device permits Hawking to communicate via emails, write books, and browse the Internet using only his cheek muscle.

In the last several years, Hawking's health has continued to decline as he was no longer able to drive his wheelchair independently in 2009 and soon required a ventilator at all times. But in 2012, on his 70th birthday, Hawking meet a group of specialists from Intel who wanted to apply state of the art technology to allow Hawking extended communication options.

Wheelchairs are designed differently depending upon the need in different environments. The wheel size, shape and configuration are based on surface needs. Size of the wheels is also a consideration for ease of using the wheelchair as well as the overall weight of the chair. The decision regarding power versus manpower is based upon the expense, weight, mobility needs, safety, physical limitations and exercise tolerance.

Wheelchair considerations:

- Folding and lifting the chair
- Seat width
- Seat depth
- Foot rest height
- Backrest
- Armrests

- Seatbelt
- Wheelchair cushion

Wheelchair accessibility to the world has been developed by the disability rights movement and the Americans with Disabilities Act of 1990 (ADA). By this mandate, in the United States the principle of universal design must accommodate all persons regardless of disability and enable access to all parts of society including public transportation and buildings.

Adaptations have included:

- Ramps
- Elevators
- Power doors
- Lowered fixtures (sinks, water fountains, counter tops)
- Toilets with safety devices
- Doorways
- Showers
- Wet rooms
- Public transportation accommodations

Standards for wheelchairs have also been established. These accommodations have also begun to spread to developed countries, while in underdeveloped and developing countries new wheelchairs are being developed.

Recently the development of the exoskeleton or bionic suit has enabled wheelchair dependent individuals to stand up and walk over ground with a natural, full weight-bearing, reciprocal gait. Walking is achieved by the user shifting weight, which activates sensors and initiates a step. Battery-powered motors mobilize the legs. This exoskeleton has applications for those patients who suffer from paralysis, deficits in arm strength and inability to walk. It helps patients relearn proper step patterns and weight shifts. Appropriate patients are those who suffered from stroke, spinal cord injury, traumatic brain injury or other conditions that limit the ability to walk.

Now we can take weak or deconditioned patients and begin to mobilize them in this assisted device. The suit educates while recovery progresses and has the ability to retrain muscle memory. These robotic exoskeletons now provide additional hope to those who suffer from inability to ambulate.

The first exoskeleton like device was developed in 1890 by a Russian named Nicholas Yagn. The first true exoskeleton, however, was developed by General Electric and the United States military in the 1960s. The suits were originally designed so a soldier could carry heavier objects during activities. They have subsequently been applied to the areas of stroke and spinal cord injury and are now commonly regarded as a wearable robot. There have been many developmental issues that cause limitations and they include power supply, skeleton, actuators, joint flexibility, power control and modulation, detection of unsafe motions, pinching, and adaptation regarding size of the individual wearing this device. Though the exoskeleton continues to be a work in progress, it still offers an additional hope for those who suffer and the potential for recovery.

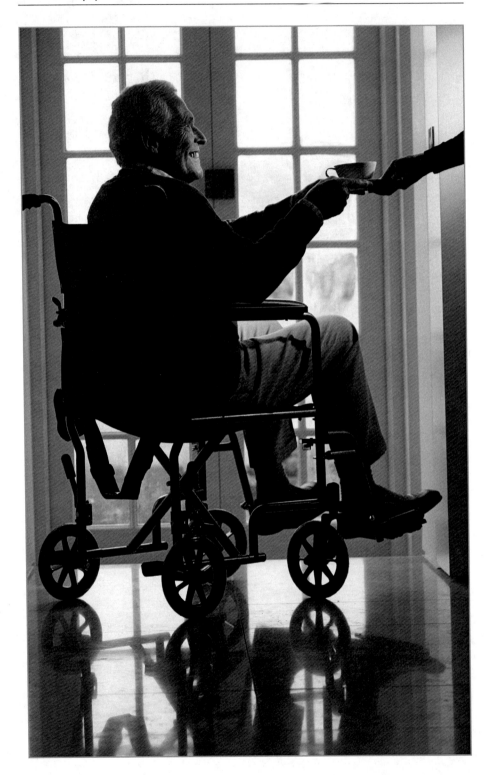

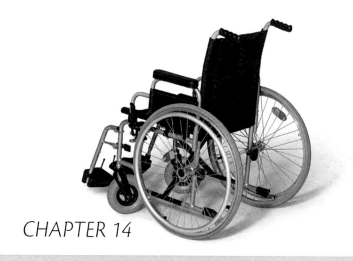

CHAPTER 14

THE MENTAL GAME

Life is filled with many adversities. In order to live an active fulfilled life sometimes one must learn to endure and strive for improvement. Just look at Christopher Reeve and Governor Greg Abbott who in spite of quadriplegia and paraplegia respectively were able to make huge contributions to society.

CASE STUDY: GOVERNOR GREGG ABBOTT

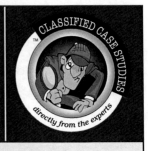

Governor Greg Abbott is an American lawyer and politician who is currently serving as the 48th Governor of Texas. He is also a partially paralyzed paraplegic who became wheelchair bound when an oak tree fell on him while he was running, following a storm in 1984.

He subsequently underwent surgery, extensive rehabilitation and is currently wheelchair dependent. He announced his gubernatorial campaign on the 29th anniversary of his accident. "Some politicians talk about having a steel spine. I actually have one," he said.

Despite the loss of his legs, Abbott was determined to rebuild himself physically. To do this, he would roll up an eight-story parking garage, spending hours going up the ramps. His commitment to strengthening the aspects of his body that he could after the accident likely served to keep him help and build his resiliency.

Upon winning his election, he became the first elected governor to sit in a wheelchair since George Wallace of Alabama in 1982. Rather than keeping his disability hidden like FDR, he leveraged it as a sign of strengths and endurance in his campaign. He believes he is proof that being confined to a wheelchair doesn't have to limit an individual's possibilities and finds serving in elected office as validation of his belief system.

Elisabeth Kübler-Ross wrote about the five stages of death and dying. Those five stages include denial, anger, bargaining, depression and acceptance. Everyone who suffers a loss goes through the stages in their own specific way. Their grief is individual with its own individual timeline. But the decision is clear.

If you had the choice between life or death, ability or disability, what would you choose? **The human condition is one of strug-**

gle, failure, reinvention and success. This is the story of the human will to adapt. So how do we as humans face seemingly insurmountable adversities and learn to adapt?

First of all adaptation is a reflection of survival of the fittest. The development of adaptive plasticity or the ability to react to environmental challenges determines survival. Thus adaptation is a process of development of a mental state rather than the actual physical body. The ability to accept change and form adaptations for survival is based on a strong will, genetic background and a supportive environment.

Choosing ability over the acceptance of disability requires a strong mind, support mechanism, supportive environment and the desire for survival.

The Move It Program

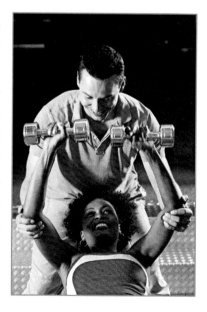

The move it program is designed to be proactive, so you can feel better and be healthy. Arthritis affects cartilage, which is the smooth protective tissue that covers bones where they meet and allows them to glide and move easily. When you develop arthritis, the cartilage wears away, the bone rubs together, and it makes it hard to move. When joints do not move, the tendons and muscles around the joint stiffen and become painful when the joint is moved.

In order to get stronger and move better after injury, you must focus on four types of exercise: muscle strengthening, core strengthening, aerobics and flexibility. To achieve the best results from your time and effort, always warm up and cool down for any kind of exercise. Take small steps when starting, gradually building up your exercise routine.

Strengthening exercises should be done three days/week and in 15–30 minute sessions. Flexibility stretches should be done seven days/week for five minutes/day. Aerobics/cardio activity should be done for five to 30 minutes, three days/week. You can progress to a daily routine as you get healthier. Aerobic exercise (walking, dancing, exercise class, etc.) is usually weight-bearing exercise. Non-weight-bearing exercise (swimming, water aerobics, and bike riding) are for those patients who are weight-bearing intolerant so they can get started and gradually work up to weight-bearing exercise.

Office workers are generally sedentary during the workday. It is well known that a sedentary lifestyle has an increased risk for diabetes, obesity, cancer, heart disease and generally a lower than average life expectancy. In order for office workers to get more physical activity during their workday the desk treadmill was developed. The thought process is that this exercise machine will increase productivity and health. Studies have shown that the treadmill user may burn 100–130 calories per hour at speeds slower than 2 miles per hour, so weight loss is a side benefit of the use of the walking treadmill desk. The treadmill desk is not intended for aerobic exercise but rather to increase the metabolism of the user over their normal basal metabolic rate. Users of the treadmill desk should not give up their traditional desk and chair, but should consider alternating between the sitting and walking desks.

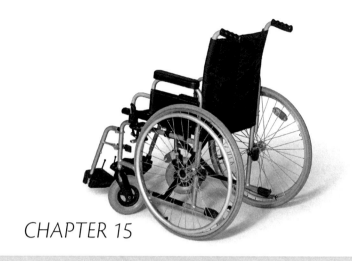

CHAPTER 15

THE FUTURE

S
ome would say that the golden era of spine care has passed. After 30 years of practice as an orthopedic surgeon specializing in spine care I beg to differ. All of medicine is currently undergoing a reorganization phase similar to other industries. Currently there is a glut of providers, hospitals, medical manufacturers and pharmaceutical companies all competing for a slowly expanding population. Insurance companies and government have decreased reimbursement rates and increased deductibles in order to slow consumption. In spite of all this, our population is healthier than it has ever been and life expectancies have been extended at least two decades for both males and females. So the evolution of spine care, new technology, techniques and treatment has led to a more active and productive population.

Newer nonoperative treatment techniques including specific exercise programs, better nutrition, nutritional supplements, smoking cessation, low-level laser therapy and injury prevention programs have been more effective in avoiding injury and aiding the body's ability to recover itself. Recent evaluation of embryonic or adult stem cell therapy is underway. New biopharmaceuticals are showing promise for medical treatment.

With the introduction of technology such as digital imaging and electronic medical records, we can now record and transmit medical information anywhere around the world. Healthcare trackers linked to your cellphone can assess your medical condition, record and even offer advice about potentially detrimental conditions.

Diagnostic imaging has progressed from simple plain X-rays to more advanced noninvasive imaging such as magnetic resonance imaging (MRI) and positron emission tomography (PET), which can provide images of the body as well as determine how a condition is developing. Also the development of advanced intraoperative imaging has opened the door to more precise implantation of spinal devices.

Surgery has progressed from large incisions requiring lengthy hospital stays to small incisions requiring either outpatient or one- to two-day hospital stays. These surgeries have been aided by the evolution of spinal instrumentation from wires to Harrington rods, pedicle screw fixation, interbody devices, artificial disc replacements, techniques for developing harvesting of autograft, and bone graft substitutes. The development of blood banks, intraoperative neurological monitoring, perioperative antibiotics, and accelerated postoperative recovery programs have led the way for patients to have more complete surgical procedures and shorter hospital stays with fewer complications. Postoperative bracing has allowed for the avoidance of prolonged bed rest, earlier mobilization and fewer complications. The exoskeleton can now elevate the wheelchair dependent to ambulatory status for exercise and limited function.

In retrospect, the past 30 years have been an extremely exciting time to provide spine care and the future seems even brighter in spite of differing opinions. I look forward to what new discoveries are coming next.

Before you wear out your back and need a spinal transplantation please remember that there is no such thing as a spinal transplant at this time. Spinal physicians can repair and replace damaged areas of the spine but they are unable to replace the entire spine. And the same applies for brain injuries. So prevention of injury, overuse and abuse is key.

By addressing some of the risk factors of spine pain one may lower the risk of developing spine pain. Treating medical problems early, such as hypertension, may prevent a stroke in the future.

Prevention usually involves daily exercise, taking your prescribed medication, stopping smoking, controlling your weight, practicing proper lifting, wearing your seatbelt and wearing your helmet if you ride a motorcycle.

We hope that by actively engaging in prevention we will have fewer wheelchairs used in this country and that more people will participate in self care in order to lead a more active and productive life.

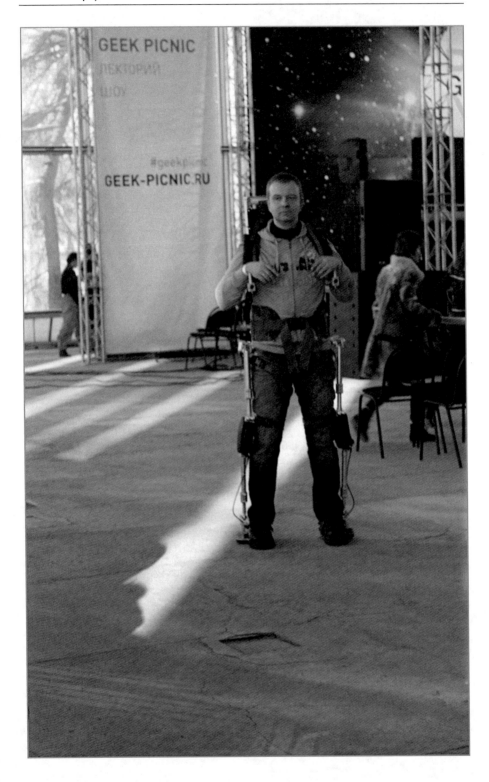

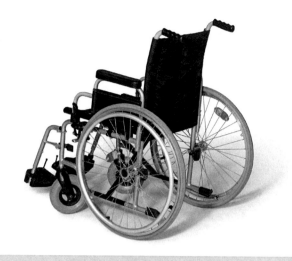

GLOSSARY

Ablation – The removal of an organ, abnormal growth or harmful area from the body by a mechanical means

Accelerated Postoperative Recovery (APR) – Program of treatment used after surgery to accelerate recovery and decrease complications

Accelerated recovery program – Technique used to enhance the body's ability to recover itself after injury, illness or surgery

Acquired immune deficiency syndrome (AIDS) – A condition caused by an infection from the human immunodeficiency virus (HIV)

Activities of daily living (ADLs) – Refers to people's daily self-care activities

Addison's disease – A chronic condition brought on by the failure of the adrenal glands

Anabolic steroids – Synthetic derivatives of the male hormone testosterone

Apoptosis – A natural process of self-destruction of a cell, which is also known as programmed cell death

Atherosclerosis – The buildup of fats, cholesterol and other substances in and on your artery walls, or plaque, that results in the restriction of blood flow

Autonomic dysreflexia (hyperreflexia) – A reaction of the autonomic or involuntary nervous system to overstimulation that is a potentially life-threatening condition

Autonomic nervous system – Division of peripheral nervous system that controls the function of internal organs

Beta-endorphin – A potent hormone that is released by the body's anterior pituitary gland in response to pain, trauma, exercise or other forms of stress and is known as the body's own pain killer

Blastocyte – An undifferentiated embryonic cell. Cells that are derived from the inner cell mass of the blastocyst are known as embryonic stem cells

Body mass index (BMI) – A formula used to calculate a person's body fat content based on his or her weight and height

Calorie – A unit of food energy that is approximately the amount of energy needed to raise the temperature of 1 kg of water by 1 C

Caudal – The anatomic route meaning inferior or below another structure in order to gain access to an anatomic area

Cell senescence – The gradual deterioration or aging of a cell

Cerebrovascular accident (CVA) – The sudden death of brain cells due to a lack of oxygen when the blood flow to the brain is impaired by either blockage or rupture of an artery in the brain. More commonly known as a stroke.

Complete injury – Where there is a total lack of sensory and motor function below the level of injury

Contamination – The unwanted pollution of something by another substance

Corticotropin-releasing hormone – A peptide hormone involved in the stress response

Cortisol – A steroid hormone produced by the adrenal cortex and released by the body in response to stress and low blood glucose

Creatine – A nitrogenous organic acid that helps to supply energy to all cells in the body, especially muscle, as it increases the formation of adenosine triphosphate (ATP)

CT scan – Computed tomography scan

Deep vein thrombosis (DVT) – A condition where a blood clot forms in a vein deep inside a part of the body

Disability – A consequence of an impairment that may be physical, cognitive, mental, sensory, emotional, developmental or some combination of these

Discectomy – The surgical removal of a herniated disc that is putting pressure on a spinal nerve or the spinal cord

Doctor – The holder of an accredited doctoral graduate degree

Dual X-ray absorbtiometry (DXA) – The preferred technique for measuring bone mineral density or soft bone

Durotomy – The incision of the dura mater or the tissue surrounding the spinal cord or nerve root

EMG – Electromyography study

Epidural Steroid Injection (ESI) – A medical route of administration where a drug or medicine is placed above the dura where the membrane surrounding the spinal cord or nerve

Epithelialization – A component of wound healing where there is a growth of epithelial or skin cells over an injured area

Fibroblastic repair – A phase in wound healing where fibroblast cells begin activity leading to scar formation

Foraminotomy – The enlargement of the spinal nerve hole or foramina in order to relieve pressure on a spinal nerve

Fragility fracture – Any fall from a standing height or less that results in a fracture

Handicap – A disadvantage that makes achievement unusually difficult. It results when a disability or impairment limits or prevents the fulfillment of a role

Heat exhaustion – A heat-related illness that occurs after exposure to high temperature

Heatstroke – A condition caused by your body overheating due to prolonged exposure to a high temperature and represents a medical emergency

Hibiclens (Mölnlycke Health Care, Gothenburg, Sweden) – A 4 percent chlorhexidine gluconate solution (CHG) that acts as an antiseptic and antimicrobial skin cleanser used to prevent infection

Human growth hormone (HGH) – Produced in the pituitary gland and helps to regulate body composition, body fluids, muscle and bone growth, sugar and fat metabolism, and possibly heart function; used by some as a performance-enhancing drug to build muscle, improve athletic performance and decrease aging

Hypermetabolism – The body's state of an increased rate of metabolic activity

Hypometabolism – The body's state of decreased rate of metabolic activity

Impact (Nestlé Health Sciences) – A nutritional supplement with arginine, omega-3 fatty acids and nucleotides to help meet the immune response in a postoperative or post injury requirement need

Impairment – A medical evaluation that determines the state of being diminished, weakened or damaged either physically or mentally

Incomplete injury – Where the ability of the spinal cord to convey messages to and from the brain is not completely lost

Inflammation – The process where the white blood cells and tissue fluids are delivered to an injured tissue

Insulin-like growth factor-1 (IGF-1) – A protein hormone necessary for proper growth in children and used by athletes to accelerate recover, but significantly increases the risk of cancer development

Interspinous device – A new spinal implant that is placed between the vertebral bodies spinous processes for the treatment of lumbar spinal degenerative disease

Laminectomy – The surgical removal of the bony posterior arch of a spinal vertebra in order to access the spinal canal

Laminotomy – The partial removal of the bony posterior arch of the spinal vertebra in order to access the spinal canal

Level of injury – The determination by a physician of the location of the spinal cord injury

LLLT – Low-level laser therapy

MEP – Motor evoked potentials

Metabolic equivalent of tasks (METs) – The metabolic unit used to quantify the intensity of physical activity; defined as the ratio of the metabolic rate during exercise to the metabolic rate at rest

Microdiscectomy – Or microdecompression spine surgery, is where through a small incision a small amount of bone may be removed from the spine in order to gain access and relieve pressure on a nerve

Morbid obesity – When excess body fat becomes a danger to your overall health

MRI – Magnetic resonance imaging

NCV - Nerve conduction velocity study

Neurogenic shock – The physiological response to shock that results in low blood pressure, occasionally a slowed heart rate and is attributed to the disruption of the autonomic pathways within the spinal cord

Nonsteroidal anti-inflammatory drug (NSAIDS) – A class of drugs that provides pain-killing, fever-reducing, and anti-inflammatory effects

Obesity – A condition where you have too much body fat for your height or have an elevated body mass index (BMI)

Osteoarthritis – The "wear and tear" arthritis; occurs when the protective cartilage on the ends of the bones wears down over time

Osteopenia – A mild thinning of bone mass that weakens bone structure

Osteoporosis – A marked thinning of bone mass that weakens bone structure

Paraplegia – An impairment in the motor or sensory function to the lower extremities

Phantom pain – A perception experienced relating to a limb or organ that is not physically part of your body

Photobiomodulation – Also known as low-level laser therapy, is the exposure of a low-level laser light or light emitting diode that stimulates cellular function leading to a beneficial clinical effect

Pilates – A physical fitness system developed by Joseph Pilates that is intended to strengthen the body and mind

Platelet-rich plasma (PRP) – Blood plasma that has been enriched with platelets and is used to concentrate growth factors that are important in the healing of injuries

Pronation – A rotation of the hand or foot to a position of either palm or sole down, respectively

Pulmonary embolism (PE) – A blood clot that has migrated to the lungs; results in restricted blood flow inside the lungs, and results in poor oxygen exchange

Quadriplegia – An impairment in the motor or sensory function to the upper and lower extremities

Radiculopathy – A pinched nerve in the spine

RICE principle – The immediate treatment of any soft tissue injury or skeletal muscle injury through rest, ice, compression and elevation

SOMI – Suboccipital mandibular orthosis

Spinal cord injury – Any damage to the spinal cord or nerves that causes changes in sensation, strength or other body functions

Spinal fusion – A surgery to permanently connect two or more spinal vertebra so there is no movement

Spinal shock – A term that relates to the loss of all neurological activity, including loss of motor, sensory, reflex and autonomic function below the level of injury

Spondylolisthesis – A condition of the spine where one bone slides forward over another bone below it

SSEP – Somatosensory evoked potentials

Stem cell – An undifferentiated, or blank, cell that has the potential to develop into other cells serving many different functions in many parts of the body

Supination – A rotation of the hand or foot to a position of either palm or sole up, respectively

TENS – Transcutaneous electrical nerve stimulation

Transforaminal – Route going through a foramen of the spine

Transitional mobility assister – Any device that allows a more efficient use of energy for locomotion (cane, crutches, wheelchair, scooter, etc.)

Translaminar – Route going across or through a lamina of the spine

U.S. Food and Drug administration (FDA) – A federal agency of the United States Department of Health and Human Services that is responsible for protecting the public health by regulating food, dietary supplements, tobacco, prescription and over-the-counter pharmaceutical medications, vaccines, blood transfusions, biopharmaceuticals, medical devices, animal foods and feed, veterinary products, and electromagnetic radiation emitting devices

Vertebrectomy – The removal of a spinal vertebra

Vitamin – An organic compound or vital nutrient that the body requires in a limited amount

Yoga – A physical, mental and spiritual practice that originated in India

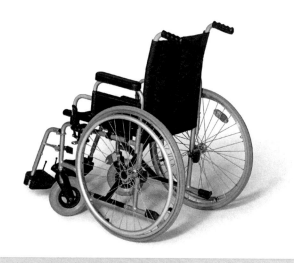

REFERENCES

Anderson, M., S. Hall and M. Martin. *Sports Injury Management*. 2nd ed. Philadelphia: Lippincott Williams and Wilkins, 2000. Print.

"Ankle Sprains: How to Speed Your Recovery." *Down East Orthopedics*. American Orthopaedic Society for Sports Medicine, 2008. Web. **www.downeastorthopedics.com/assets/Ankle-Sprains.pdf**.

Arden, C.L., N. F. Taylor, J.A. Feller and K.E. Webster. " A systematic review of psychological factors associated with returning to sports following injury." *British Journal of Sports Medicine* 47 (2013): 1120-1126.

Berish, Amy, "FDR and Polio." Franklin D. Roosevelt Presidential Library and Museum, 2014. Web. **www.fdrlibrary. marist.edu/aboutfdr/polio.html**.

Bleeker, Michiel WP, et al. "Vascular adaptation to deconditioning and the effect of an exercise countermeasure: results of the Berlin Bed Rest study." *Journal of Applied Physiology* 99.4 (2005): 1293-1300.

Bohn, Kevin and Ashley Killough, "Former President George H. W. Bush in 'fair condition'" CNN,16 July 2015. Web. **www.cnn. com/2015/07/15/politics/bush-41-hospital-fall-maine**.

Bahr, Roald and Sverre Maehlum. *Clinical Guide to Sports Injuries*. Champaign: Human Kinetics, 2004. Print.

Campbell, Barbara J. "Calcium, Nutrition, and Bone Health." Orthoinfo. AAOS, July 2012. Web. **http://orthoinfo.aaos.org/ topic.cfm?topic=A00317**.

"Christopher Reeve: Biography." Christopher & Dana Reeve Foundation. Web. **www.christopherreeve.org/site/c. ddJFKRNoFiG/b.4431483**.

Cotler, H.B. "A NASA discovery has current applications in orthopedics." *Current Orthopaedic Practice* 26.1 (2015): 72-74.

Cotler, H.B., R.T. Chow, M.R. Hamblin and J. Carroll. "The use of low level laser therapy (LLLT) for musculoskeletal pain." *MOJ Orthopedics & Rheumatology* 2.5 (2015): 1-8.

Crane, Kristine. "Enhanced recovery: improving patient surgical experience." U.S. News and World Report, 4 Feb. 2015. Web. **http://health.usnews.com/health-news/patient-advice/ articles/2015/02/04/enhanced-recovery-improving-patients- surgical-experience**.

Dooley, Erin, "George H. W. Bush Marks 90th Birthday by Skydiving," ABC News, 12 June 2014. Web. **http://abcnews. go.com/Politics/george-bush-marks-90th-birthday-skydiving/ story?id=24103264**.

Eisenbraun, Karen, "Elizabeth Taylor – A Life of Pain and Multiple Surgeries," VacuPractor, 14 May 2011. Web. **www.vacupractor.com/famous-people/elizabeth-taylor-a-life-of-pain-and-multiple-surgeries**.

Garbutt, G., M.G. Boocock, T. Reilly and J.D. Troup. "Running speed and spinal shrinkage in runners with and without back pain." *Medicine & Science in Sports & Exercise* 22.6 (1990): 769-772.

Giza, Christopher C. and David A. Hovda, "The Neurometabolic Cascade of Concussion." *Journal of Athletic Training* 36.3 (2001): 228-235.

Hagen, K.B., G. Jamtvedt, G. Hilde and M.F. Winnem. "The updated Cochrane review of bed rest for low back pain and sciatica." *Spine (Phila Pa 1976)* 30.5 (2005): 542-546. PubMed 9971865.

Harte, J.L., G.H. Eifert and R. Smith. "The effect of running and meditation on beta-endorphin, corticotropin-releasing hormone and cortisol in plasma, and on mood." *Biological Psychology* 40.3 (1995): 251-265.

Hetzel, Megan. "570-Pound Man Commits to Finishing a 5K Per Month in 2015," Runner's World, 20 March 2015. **www.runnersworld.com/newswire/570-pound-man-commits-to-finishing-a-5k-per-month-in-2015**.

Hubbard, T.J. and C.R. Denegar. "Does cryotherapy improve outcomes with soft tissue injury?" *Journal of Athletic Training* 39.3 (2004): 278-279.

Hupin, D., et al. "Even low dose to moderate to vigorous physical activity reduces mortality by 22% in adults aged equal to or greater than 60 years: a systematic review and meta-analysis." *British Journal of Sports Medicine* doi:10.1136/bjsports-2014-094306.

Hutchinson, A. "Fitness: Ice baths, antioxidant supplements not always the best route to recovery." The Globe and Mail, 23 Aug. 2015. Web. **www.theglobeandmail.com/life/health-and-fitness/ fitness/ice-baths-antioxidant-supplements-not-always-the- best-route-to-recovery/article26052576.**

Inskeep, Steve, "Former President George H.W. Bush Throws Out First Pitch," NPR, 12 Oct. 2015. Web. **www.npr. org/2015/10/12/447911238/former-president-george-h-w-bush- throws-out-first-pitch.**

Jackson, David, "George H.W. Bush talks about mobility problems." USA Today, 13 July 2012. Web. **http://content. usatoday.com/communities/theoval/post/2012/07/hw-bush- talks-about-mobility-problems/1#.VpcZm5OAOko.**

Kelly, Frank B. "Platelet-Rich Plasma (PRP)." OrthoInfo. AAOS, Sept. 2011. Web. **http://orthoinfo.aaos.org/topic. cfm?topic=A00648.**

Kübler-Ross, Elisabeth. *On Death and Dying.* London: Routledge, 1969. Print.

Kübler-Ross, Elisabeth and David Kessler. *On Grief and Grieving: Finding the Meaning of Grief Through the Five Stages of Loss.* New York: Scribner, 2005. Print.

LaPlante, Mitchell P. and D. Carlson. "Disability in the United States: Prevalence and causes, 1992." *Disability Statistics Report,* 7. Washington, D.C.: U.S. Department of Education, National Institute on Disability and Rehabilitation Research (1996).

LaPlante, Mitchell P., G.E. Hendershot and A.J. Moss. "Assistive Technology Devices and Home Accessibility Features: Prevalence, Payment, Needs and Trends." *Advance Data from Vital and Health Statistics* 217 (1992). Hyattsville, Maryland: National Center for Health Statistics.

Manini, T.M., et al. "Daily activity energy expenditure and mortality among older adults." *Journal of the American Medical Association* 296.2 (2006): 171-179.

McCoy, Terrence. "Once the world's heaviest man, Manuel Uribe dies." The Washington Post, 27 May 2014. Web. **www. washingtonpost.com/news/morning-mix/wp/2014/05/27/once-the-worlds-heaviest-man-manuel-uribe-dies**.

Medeiros, Joao. "How Intel Gave Stephen Hawking a Voice." Wired, 13 Jan. 2015. Web. **www.wired.com/2015/01/intel-gave-stephen-hawking-voice**.

"National Health Interview Survey on Disability." *Centers for Disease Control and Prevention*. USA.gov, 1994. Web. **www.cdc. gov/nchs/nhis/nhis_disability.htm**.

Neumann, Janice. "For seniors, any exercise may be better than none." Reuters, 21 Aug. 2015. Web. **www. reuters.com/article/us-health-elderly-fitness-mortality-idUSKCN0QQ1M620150821**.

Ogden C.L., M.D. Carroll, B.K. Kit and F.M. Flegal. "Prevalence of childhood and adult obesity in the United States." *The Journal of the American Medical Association* 311.8 (2014): 806-814.

Oldmeadow, L.B., E.R. Edwards, L.A. Kimmel, et al. "No rest for the wounded: early ambulation after hip surgery accelerates recovery." *ANZ Journal of Surgery* 76.7 (2006): 607-611. PubMed #16813627.

Patrick, C.A., et al. "Lack of effectiveness of bed rest for sciatica." *The New England Journal of Medicine* 340.6 (1999): 418-423. PubMed#9971865.

Romano, Lois, "Riding Accident Paralyzes Actor Christopher Reeve," The Washington Post, 1 June 1995. Web. **www. washingtonpost.com/wp-dyn/articles/A99660-1995Jun1.html**.

Russell, J.N., G.E. Hendershott, F. LeClere, L.J. Howie and M. Adler. "Trends and differential use of assistive technology devices: United States, 1994." *Advance Data from Vital and Health Statistics* 292. Hyattsville, Maryland: National Center for Health Statistics, 1997.

Sorrenti, S.J. "Achilles tendon rupture: effective early mobilization in rehabilitation after surgical repair." *Foot & Ankle International* 27.6 (2006): 407-410. PubMed#16764705.

Storrs, Carina. "Is Platelet-Rich Plasma and Effective Healing Therapy?" Scientific American, 18 Dec. 2009. Web. www. scientificamerican.com/article/platelet-rich-plasma-therapy-dennis-cardone-sports-medicine-injury.

Vigelsoe, Andreas, et al. "Six weeks' aerobic training after two weeks' immobilization restores leg lean mass and aerobic capacity but does not fully rehabilitate leg strength in young and older men." *Journal of Rehabilitation Medicine* (2015) doi: 10.2340/16501977-1961.

Weiner, Rachel, "Five things to know about Greg Abbott." The Washington Post, 15 July 2013. Web. **www.washingtonpost. com/news/the-fix/wp/2013/07/15/five-things-to-know-about-greg-abbott**.

Weinstein, James N., et al. "Surgical versus Non-Operative Treatment for Lumbar Spinal Stenosis Four-Year Results of the Spine Patient Outcome Research Trial (SPORT)." *Spine* (Phila Pa 1976) 35.14 (2010): 1329-1338.

Zhang, Yuqing and Joanne M. Jordan. "Epidemiology of osteoarthritis." *Clinics in Geriatric Medicine* 26.3 (2010): 355-369.

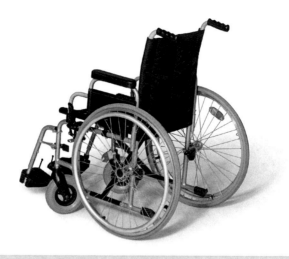

AUTHOR BIOGRAPHY

H oward B. Cotler, MD, FACS, FAAOS is board certified and recertified in Orthopedic Surgery. He is a fellow of the American Academy of Orthopedic Surgery and the American College of Surgeons. He received his medical degree in 1979 from Jefferson Medical College of Thomas Jefferson University in Philadelphia. In 1980, Dr. Cotler completed his surgical internship at Grady Memorial Hospital/ Emory University in Atlanta. In 1984, he completed his orthopedic residency at Thomas Jefferson University Hospital.

Dr. Cotler subsequently pursued advanced training in spine through two fellowships: one in acute spinal cord injury surgery with Northwestern University in Chicago in 1984 and another in Orthopedic Traumatology with Harborview Medical Center/ University of Washington in Seattle in 1985. From 1985 to 1990,

Dr. Cotler had both a clinical practice and an academic appointment at the University of Texas Medical School in Houston. In 1990, he became a founding partner and medical director for the Texas Back Institute of Houston. He was clinical associate professor of Orthopedic Surgery at the University of Texas Medical School in Houston. In 1995 Dr. Cotler founded Gulf Coast Spine Care Limited PA.

If you like this book, you can find more information at www.gulfcoastspinecare.com and follow Dr. Cotler on Twitter, LinkedIn and Facebook.

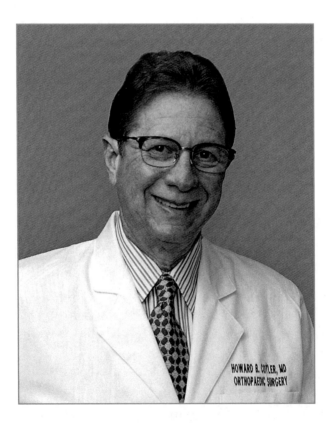

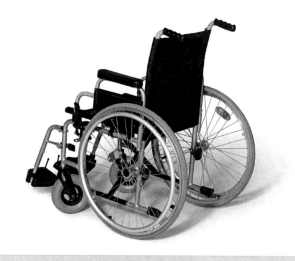

INDEX

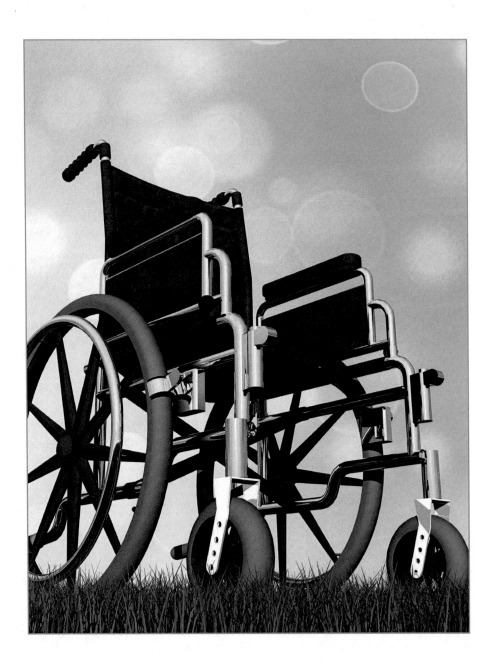